LEADING DEPARTMENT EXCELLENCE

Achieve the Robust Academic Health Center

RICHARD I. BURTON, MD

ISBN: 1495314987
ISBN 13: 9781495314988
Library of Congress Control Number: 2014901691
CreateSpace Independent Publishing Platform
North Charleston, South Carolina

Contents

Section VI: Case Studies 313

These twelve case studies each present the "facts of the case" but not the discussion and possible answers. They are to be used to foster thoughts and/or discussions for those individuals who might use this book as a "manual" for a mentoring program for new and established Chairs.

Some Items to Consider for Sample Prototype Documents

To Peggy, whose love, support, wisdom, understanding, patience, and energy have encouraged and sustained me in my endeavors for more than fifty years.

Introduction

Justification for this document: Why write this book? What precipitated this effort?

To be Chair of an academic Department in an Academic Health Center (AHC) is an honor, carries much responsibility, and will make a real difference in the lives and careers of other AHC leaders, faculty, fellows, residents, students, and staff. To be a Chair can be most gratifying. Many skills are needed to nurture the careers of others, to foster great academic programs (research, patient care, education), and to create new product and service lines.

To accomplish such is great fun and truly enjoyable. The author knows this well from having been the Chair of three different Departments in the same AHC over many years.

Academic Health Centers (AHCs) are very complex in organizational structure. The goal/mission/vision is multifaceted: a) delivering the best possible care both to the individually afflicted patient and to afflicted populations; b) educating the present and future generation of healthcare professionals; c) educating current and future research scientists; d) conducting clinical, basic, and translational research; and e) establishing community outreach, including the education of the public at large about health issues to foster the health of the community. All of these have the targeted intent of advancing medical knowledge for the betterment of patient care and population health in future generations. However, "no money, no mission." For the AHC to be viable for the present and the future, superb organization and financial management are essential.

> *"It always seems impossible until it's done."*
> —NELSON MANDELA

In the face of these challenges, it must be noted that:

1) Most new Chairs are poorly prepared for the tasks and challenges that await them. These problems that need to be addressed should not surprise anyone who has considered the following. Academic faculty in AHCs develop prowess in clinical, research, and/or teaching spheres, but have limited administrative experience. The most accomplished of these individuals bubble up to the top as potential Chair candidates at either their own or another AHC. Suddenly these accomplished individuals are thrust into a new realm. Although prior traditional academic skill sets give these new Chairs academic credibility, these new Chairs need instant broad-ranging talents/skills that they often never previously needed and might not have. Thus, not infrequently emerges the potential case of the "fatal flaw" in which the new Chair has a great academic track record and an extraordinarily high IQ, yet also has poor administrative skills/knowledge and/or undeveloped emotional intelligence.

The tradition is that Chairs of clinical Departments must sit comfortably on a **three**-legged stool—patient care, research, and education. The recently added **fourth** leg is community outreach and population health. Except for the extraordinary individual, most clinical Chairs sit firmly on two of the traditional three, but *MUST* appreciate the third and fourth, and be certain that the Department addresses all four missions. For basic science Chairs, the stool traditionally must have two solid legs---education and research.

There is now for all Chairs, basic science and clinical, an essential additional leg on the stool—executive administrative leadership, including emotional intelligence. This is an absolutely key additional **fifth** leg of the stool for clinical Chairs and the **third** leg of the stool for basic science Chairs. Without this additional leg, the stool will come tumbling down. For many new Chairs (and some existing Chairs), this leg is often weak or even missing.

2) It is essential that Chairs and/or Center Directors be MD, DO, or MD/ PhD for clinical Departments and PhD or PhD/MD for basic science Departments. Those backgrounds are prerequisites and irreplaceable for: a) credibility with peers and faculty; b) identification, assessment, strategies, and delivery of all the "product lines"; and c) acute awareness of opportunities and threats within his/her clinical and/or scientific expertise. That said, these Chair leaders must learn new skill sets, and most often will need advice from those with business and legal backgrounds.

The Chair can better lead when he/she measures progress. The reader is referred to Appendix D for some helpful metrics that should be tracked by the Chair leader.

A few basic definitions the author has used throughout the text:

1) The term *Chair* will be used to indicate one of several positions within the AHC.

   a) The traditional sense of the word as the Chair of an academic Department (be it clinical or basic science)

   b) The head of a large Division within a big Department

   c) The Director of a mission-focused Center

   d) The Director of a multi-Departmental "product"

2) Consistent with that use of the term *Chair*, the term *Department* will indicate:

   a) The traditional academic Department

   b) A large Division within a big traditional Department

c) A mission-focused Center

d) A multi-Departmental "product line"

3) To be gender sensitive, the term *he/she* will be used.

4) *Senior Leadership* will vary from one AHC to another, but the term is intended, as applicable, to include the Chief Executive Officer (may include in some AHCs a "President" or "Vice President" or "Vice Provost" titles as well), the Dean, the Director(s) of the Hospital(s), and the Chief Financial Officer (CFO). In some AHCs, this Senior Leadership group may also include the Office of Counsel, the Director of the Faculty Practice Group, and others.

> *"For the things we have to learn before we can do them, we learn by doing them."*
>
> —ARISTOTLE

This book is written for:

1) New Chairs looking for guidance

2) Late-middle and senior faculty seeking to be a Chair

3) Younger faculty who wonder what it's like to be a Chair and what they might need to do now to begin to position themselves for consideration in the future

4) Some established Chairs, who may find valuable guidance in certain chapters

The conundrums facing Chairs and those in similar positions:

1) How to balance the goals and needs of the Department with those of the AHC

2) How to advocate for AHC and at the same time also for the Department missions and for the Department faculty

3) How to balance clinical, research, educational, and community outreach missions within the Department

4) In clinical spheres, how to balance medical care for the individual patient with the emerging concepts of "population health"

5) How to be collaborative with other Chairs and at the same time advance the goals and needs of one's own Department within the AHC mission and vision

6) How to deliver more products and more results with fewer resources, such as faculty, space, and funding

7) How to obtain and utilize financial, legal, compliance, and human resource input

How this text is to be used:

1) This is a compilation of suggestions and advice, and hopefully some wisdom, based upon the author's forty years of experience within AHCs.

2) This is very much a how-to-do-it book, not a book on theory. Generalities, such as "be diverse," "get consensus," or "be sensitive," convey obvious facts that are really not that helpful, unless one knows *how* to achieve them. This book provides the "how."

3) The established Chair will want to read selectively as it pertains to needs/questions concerning particular situations and challenges.

4) The aspiring or new Chair might find the entire text relevant.

5) Out of necessity, there is some repetition in various chapters, which will hopefully be of benefit to those reading selected chapters rather than the entire text. When considered prudent, some chapters are cross-referenced.

6) Regardless of whether the reader is interested in an aspiring, new, or established Chair role, this text will be most beneficial if used in conjunction with a formal mentoring program.

7) With the rapidly changing external environments for AHCs and with the great variations in AHC structures, much of the material is presented generically to explain how to do the task(s), "the fifty-thousand-foot view" of how. This broad view of the "how" will provide "the how framework" and then will require the reader to think and to extrapolate to the specifics of his/her AHC's unique situation(s) and challenge(s) and to the rapidly changing economic realities of clinical and research funding. Thus, the intent is that hopefully this document will survive to be useful independent of the evolution of our health-care, educational, and research AHCs.

What this text is NOT:

1) Suitable for generalized audiences, such as businesses or law firms

2) A general text on leadership training

3) Applicable to government agencies

4) A compilation of a leadership bibliography

> *"The farther backward you can look, the farther forward you are likely to see."*
> —Sir Winston Churchill

What qualifies the author to write this document?

1) Sixteen years of experience as Chair of three different Departments (Orthopaedics, Rehabilitation, Neurosurgery)

2) Residency program directorships and fellowship program directorships, spanning twenty-five years

3) Fostering of very successful Departmental programs in areas in
which he had no expertise by facilitating the successes of other faculty (sports/spine/research)

4) Several national leadership positions—including Director of the
American Board of Orthopaedic Surgery, voting representative to
the American Board of Medical Specialties (ABMS), leadership of
Conjoint Certificate of Qualification in Hand Surgery committee
from three Specialty Boards of the ABMS, presidency of a national professional organization (American Society for Surgery of the
Hand)

5) Service at an AHC for ten years as Senior Associate Dean for Academic
Affairs (responsible for advising Chairs and Center Directors; faculty discipline; Chair/Department/Center reviews; Chair searches;
conflict of interest policies and management; and administration of
all promotion, reappointment and tenure processes for decisions)

6) Professional awareness of, and concern for, how poorly most AHCs
develop a "pipeline" of potential future Chairs and leaders

The author gratefully acknowledges all that he has learned over the
past fifty years from those at the University of Rochester and in other
AHCs and professional organizations across the country. This includes
many Chairs, other academic leaders, teachers, colleagues, fellows, resi-
dents, and medical students. In particular, gratitude is extended to the
University of Rochester Medical Center (URMC) for granting me a sab-
batical to write this volume. A special thank-you goes to those in URMC
Senior Leadership—Dr. Bradford Berk, Dr. Mark Taubman, Dr. Lissa
McAnarney, and Dr. David Guzick—for their ongoing encouragement
to write this book and for their important relevant insights. Dr. Regis
O'Keefe, Dr. Steven Dewhurst, Dr. Robert Holloway, Dr. Jeffrey Lyness,
Gunta Liders, and Diane Caselli have been very generous and helpful

with valuable suggestions for this book. Two quiet heroes have been Lori McBride for staff support and Jason Merrill for computer and technical expertise.

> *"If you want to be successful, it's just this simple. Know what you are doing. Love what you are doing. And believe in what you are doing."*
> —WILL ROGERS

The author's intent with this book is to assist Chairs and aspiring Chairs "to know what you are doing." To "love what you are doing and believe in what you are doing" will be the responsibility of the reader.

. . . .

Be a Leader.
Make a Difference.
Enjoy!

. . . .

SECTION I

Chair Leadership in the Academic Health Center (AHC)

CHAPTER 1
....

General Observations and Pearls of Wisdom on Leadership within the Academic Health Center (AHC)

"His leadership is such that he doesn't get people to follow him; he gets people to join him."
—NFL ALL-PRO STEVE TASKER, DESCRIBING COACH MARV LEVY

What is Chair leadership? This is a question contemplated by many faculty who observe those in leadership positions, and in so doing either admire the skills and styles of the leaders they follow and hope to someday emulate them, or are distraught at what they perceive as poor, bad, or a lack of leadership. Faculty may wonder "Could I do this in the future?" or believe "I don't like what I see; I bet I could do it better." For a variety of reasons, many faculty have the potential to be future leaders—a fortunate few from the environment in which they are nourished and mentored. The majority, or perhaps all of potential future leaders, would be well-served by a focused and targeted leadership development program within the AHC. The challenges and situations of Chairs and similar leaders are unique within the AHC; thus, these Chair-leadership development programs need to be focused and tailored to those specific needs and situations.

The motivation for leadership should be the passion to improve the other faculty and the Department for the betterment of the AHC, and thereby to foster the health of the population of patients and the

individual patients for whom the Department and the AHC are responsible both today and in future years. Today's research and the current education of future clinicians and researchers will determine the health of the next generation. The passion must come from, and be for, the right reasons. The Chair who strives for and achieves the position of Chair to enhance his/her career and stature will be far less successful than the Chair who seeks to enhance the career and accomplishments of others to move forward both the Department and the AHC (see chapter 13).

This brief chapter will outline some principles and lessons learned—some the hard way, some by intuition, and some by watching others succeed while others failed due to fatal errors. This chapter will be from "the fifty-thousand-foot perspective" with some overarching concepts, pearls learned in the school of hard knocks.

Leadership does not lend itself to tidy definitions. A wise judge once proclaimed, "I cannot define it (pornography), but I know it when I see it." Leadership is obvious when seen; the more difficult the situation, the more the true leader will shine and the leadership skills be obvious. Six key broad topics will frame much of the rest of this book: a) can, and how does, one lead a group of independent thinkers?; b) leaders are not simple caretakers; c) Collins' book (6) has some essential points on successful leadership; d) Goleman (14, 15, 16) emphasizes that there are many leadership styles; e) some commonalities are exhibited by individuals trying to undermine leaders; and f) some leadership pearls on style.

1) "Leading those who may not want to be led" summarizes the challenges faced by many Chairs. Much of the rest of this book will address the following items from a variety of perspectives.

   a) Members of an academic Department, if already accomplished or with such young talent as to be on the way to becoming accomplished, will represent a group of independent thinkers. Each will have his/her own ideas on his/her role, and how the Department can/should get from point A to point B.

b) What is the role of the Department within the greater AHC, in terms of interfacing with other Chairs and with Senior Leadership?

c) Is it possible to make leadership a team sport? How can the Chair develop team consensus within the Department, develop a team approach with other Departments, and then relate to Senior Leadership as a team player?

d) Challenges will arise. Troubles will occur. Can emerging smoke be put back in the bottle? An ounce of prevention is worth a pound of cure.

2) *Leader vs. "caretaker"* is a key concept. In the successful AHC, Departments that are "cared for" are managed to maintain the status quo. This is not leadership. Failure to move forward is to go backward.

a) Leaders are people who inspire others by clearly articulating a vision of how things can be done better.

b) Good *management* controls complexity; effective *leadership* produces useful change (see Appendix D for metrics for Chair to monitor).

3) The book *Good to Great* by Collins (6) is a text that many may find helpful. In this book:

a) Many excellent points are made, especially these seven points worth contemplating as they apply to Chairs:

i) Level-five leadership can be modest/humble but still have the will, the drive, and a fearless but not reckless approach. Warren Buffett has been suggested as an excellent example.

ii) A key first step is the selection of the leader's team; then the team focuses on the "what": the mission, the vision, the goal. Jack Welch (General Electric) perceptively pointed out the wisdom for the leader to recruit people smarter and more competent than the leader.

iii) True leadership is not easy and is not for sissies. The leader must confront the brutal facts. Collins calls this the Stockdale Paradox, based upon the survival stories from American prisoners of the North Koreans during the Korean War. Stockdale confronted the reality of the brutally stark situation of the prisoners of war, not sugarcoating it. He survived.

iv) The Hedgehog Concept from Collins is important. The hedgehog in "balling up" focuses on the situation, often doing better than the fox that trots all around with diffuse, nonfocused planning and activities.

v) The leader's creation of a culture of discipline means people will act with discipline and focus but not be bound up and thwarted by the bureaucracy of a controlling system.

vi) Technology is of value only as an accelerator, a tool that, when used selectively and wisely, will be a facilitating and accelerating means to an end.

vii) The leader will foster slow, steady, relentless progress, not a single revolution.

b) With all of the wisdom in Collins' perspective, note that he missed the mark on two of the case studies he praised in his book—Circuit City and Fannie Mae. The subsequent failures of these entities highlight the difficulties inherent in trying to achieve leadership success.

i) Circuit City filed for bankruptcy in October 2008 and was liquidated January 2009.

ii) Fannie Mae (along with Fannie Mac) had a key role in the housing market collapse in 2008, and the economics of this housing situation played a key role in the subsequent collapse of the US economy.

4) **Leadership styles:**

   a) **A leader can take one of several styles** (see also chapter 13 for two basic Chair styles). Perhaps one of the most important modifiers of any type of style is what Goleman (14, 15, 16) calls "emotional intelligence," the Chair's awareness of his/her emotions linked to his/her self-control of those emotions, which can then be combined with the ability to discern what makes the other person(s) tick.

   There are pros and cons of the various leadership styles. The settings vary in which each might be effective. Importantly, no one style fits all leadership situational needs or organizational structures. To compound the situation, it can create problems and confuse the members of a team if the leader switches from one style to another. That said, there are situations and/or personalities with whom the leader has to interface, when modification of style may be the best productive course and indeed necessary. Goleman has summarized these styles:

   i) **Coercive:** "Do what I say." This is good in disaster situations, but inhibits the creativity of other faculty and does not motivate. This can work in a crisis, but not as a sustained policy.

   ii) **Authoritarian:** "Come with me." This can be good if the Department is adrift. However, this is counterproductive as it will not take advantage of the experts on the leader's team, experts who may have had experience and thus wisdom and vision that might be better than that of the leader's.

   iii) **Affiliating:** "People come first." This will make members of the Department or team "feel good," fostering harmony and a "warm fuzzy feeling," but also fostering poor performance. Team members will often get confused; incentive, focus, and targets get blurred.

iv) **Democratic:** This style of discussions and "votes" is good for flexibility and may well encourage fresh ideas. The risky downside is endless meetings and a leaderless feeling of drifting without a target or vision.

v) **Pacesetting:** This leader sets a very fast pace, a role model for all to emulate. Very talented and motivated faculty will thrive, but others who may be important but less talented will be overwhelmed.

vi) **Coaching:** This leadership style with a strong mentorship component is good for personal development of faculty, especially for faculty who are aware of their weaknesses. This is of no value for faculty who are resistant to change.

b) **There are troublesome personality types of which the leader must be aware.** These personalities rarely exist in effective leaders, but are often in those individuals who seek to undermine the leader. These are the Brinkman-Kirschner categories, cited by Cote (7). These faculty may use these techniques in meetings to be troublesome. Even more malicious can be the use of many of these personal techniques to stir up faculty discomfort and discord outside the meetings, one-on-one, and in small groups behind the leader's back. Some faculty may do this to undermine the Chair. Some will do this for personal gain. Some will do this just for the "delight" of creating problems (see also Chapters 18, 19, 22, 23, 24, 28).

i) The Steamroller or Tank: These faculty are aggressive and angry. Their interpersonal behavior risks other people getting flattened and becoming nonproductive, especially those in a reporting relationship. Faculty at the same rank will tend to "fight back." Those of higher rank tend to get angry, and those of lower rank will resent and avoid the individual.

ii) The Sniper: These faculty use sarcasm, rudeness, and eye rolls as a weapon.

iii) The Know-It-All: These faculty tend to assume/attempt to wield authority based on what they know (or mistakenly think they know). They often are intelligent experts and usually do have a lot to offer, but cannot tolerate others or situations where they get contradicted/corrected—and they have no hesitancy in going out of their way to contradict/correct others.

iv) They Think They Know It All: These faculty are different from the know-it-all, in that these individuals think knowledge in one small area makes them wise in everything; they are cocky and try to mislead/deceive/fool others into believing what they are saying, even though their "facts" are not true.

v) The Grenade: These faculty members tend to explode into uncontrolled ranting, which may or may not relate to topic or situation.

vi) The Malevolent Mentors: These are often the senior faculty members who like to stir up trouble, using junior faculty or mentees to do so, and who dispense advice that is at times good/helpful but more likely is self-serving and destructive.

vii) The Yes Person: These individuals want so much to please others that they always agree, never taking an opposing view even if that is what should be done. They will be inconsistent from one situation to the next.

viii) The Maybe Person: These are the procrastinators. They often avoid making a decision and do not want to hurt the feelings of others. This causes a lot of frustration in those with whom they work.

ix) The Blank Wall (or Nothing Person): In meetings and interactions these faculty offer blank stares and no verbal clues as to what they are thinking. Later on they can be very disruptive if behind the leader's back they revert to one of the other behaviors.

x) The No Person: These faculty will say no to new ideas, to recycled ideas, and will spread doom, gloom, and despair. These faculty will suck energy very quickly from a group or in a one-on-one interaction.

xi) The Whiner: These faculty themselves feel helpless, are easily overwhelmed by what they perceive (often falsely) to be unfair. They want everything perfect, and when not so, they whine. And these people love (and are energized by) sharing their misery with others.

"When your work speaks for itself, don't interrupt."
—HENRY J. KAISER, AMERICAN INDUSTRIALIST

5) **The dozen "pearls"** this author has found universally helpful:

a) Be calm yet passionate and inspirational, not calm and dull/sleepy.

b) When speaking, stick to the facts; do not preach.

c) There is real value in a style of genuine warmth, depth, and caring.

d) Listen well; this is very important.

e) Flexibility does *not* mean indecisive, does *not* mean inconsistent. You can listen to divergent opinions, look at all sides of an issue, and still be decisive.

f) You can change strategy, and may need to, while keeping the same goal.

g) Do not confuse hope with actual accomplishment. Hope is not a plan.

h) There are no automatic rote answers to most challenges that leaders face.

i) Self-confidence is very different from arrogance and very different from inflated self-esteem.

j) Within the AHC, the Chair must recognize that institutional vision will trump Departmental benefit, and Departmental benefit trumps individual faculty member desires.

k) One of a middle leader's true challenges is balancing the often-conflicting visions and needs of the AHC, the Department/Center/Division/Program, and groups of faculty.

l) If at all possible, the leader must seek common ground to create a win-win scenario.

. . . .

Be a Leader
Make a Difference
Enjoy!

. . . .

CHAPTER 2

Key Attributes Inherent in the Successful Chair within the Vagaries of the AHC

> *"Success is not the key to happiness. Happiness is the key to success. If you love what you are doing, you will be successful."*
>
> —ALBERT SCHWEITZER

There are strengths that the Chair, as a leader, must master. Regardless of how the AHC is organized, no matter how the AHC may reorganize, no matter how the AHC changes its goals/missions, and regardless of changes in external funding sources, these strengths must be intrinsic to the Chair. These skills are so very important and instrumental to the Chair's successes. The chapters in Section V of this book discuss in detail these skills and efforts.

> *"Knowledge without wisdom is like water in the sand."*
>
> —GUINEAN PROVERB

These internal personal attributes fall into four groups. All will be rocks of strength for the Chair and are in fact under the Chair's control regardless of the AHC structure and function, regardless of the individuals with whom the Chair interfaces, and regardless of power forces external to the AHC, such as NIH changes and third-party payor variations.

Much of Section V of this book is devoted to the development and utilization of the points in these four groups of attributes.

1) The Chair's self-perception, role, and goals:

- The Chair is the face of the Department at the AHC.

- The Chair is an important face of the AHC and the Department regionally and nationally.

- The Department is more important than the Chair.

- Department faculty's career development and successes are of more future value to the Department than those of the current Chair. The successful Chair on the national scene has an impact of one person. Multiple well-mentored and accomplished Department faculty have the impact of many individuals—a compounded national influence.

- The needs and goals of the Department must balance with and augment the needs and visions of the AHC.

- The Chair needs to lead by example with expertise in clinical care, research, and/or education.

- Based upon expertise, the Chair should set an example of national reputation, often with elected or selected national leadership positions.

2) The Chair's style:

- Stick to the facts and be consistent, calm, fair, and honest.

- Empower others.

- Praise others in public; criticize others one-on-one in private.

- Never lose one's temper; always maintain a sense of humor (clean humor!).

> *"A leader needs a true heart, a strong mind, and a great deal of courage."*
> —HARRY TRUMAN

3) The Chair's strategies should be to:

- Never lose sight of long-term goals, even if strategies to achieve those have to be modified or even changed. Be patient and persistent toward goals.

- Be vigorous, passionate, enthusiastic, and steadily committed to goals, not "hyper."

- Be imaginative and flexible (flexibility is *not* indecision).

- Align incentives, so difficult situations become "win-win."

- Do the right things for the right reasons.

- Act with dignity and integrity.

- Do not take oneself too seriously. The Chair should take the Department's mission(s)/goal(s) seriously, but not take him/herself too seriously.

- Learn to distinguish criticism of ideas/suggestions of the Chair from criticism of the person who holds the position of Chair; these also do not equate to criticism of the Chair's core value to AHC.

> *"In order to win a man to your cause, you must first reach his heart, the great high road to his reason."*
> —ABRAHAM LINCOLN

4) The Chair should be aware of whom he/she must reach, along with the key individuals with whom he/she must relate and engage in dialogue, and know how to best approach each of these individuals.

. . . .

Be a Leader
Make a Difference
Enjoy!

. . . .

CHAPTER 3

The Professionalism of the Effective Leader

> *"Always do the right thing. This will satisfy some people and astonish others."*
>
> —BENJAMIN FRANKLIN

What is a profession and how does this relate to the tone and traditions to which the middle leaders of the AHC need to aspire? *Webster's* dictionary defines a profession as "not commercial, not mechanical, not agricultural, or the like" but as "an occupation to which one devotes oneself; a calling." Professionalism must be nurtured and must survive in the face of enormous external pressures converging on the AHCs.

Professionalism, and what that implies and comprises, is a huge topic. That said, certain of the attributes inherent in professionalism are dependent on the skill sets and styles necessary to be an effective and respected leader.

In the AHC, there is the reality of "no money, no mission." This is true for the AHC as a single entity, and for each Department, Center, and Program within it. Hope is not a plan; the honest, strong desire to deliver a product, be it a research, educational, or clinical endeavor, will not happen in the absence of resources, whatever their sources might be (see Appendix D for metrics of success to measure).

The conversion of planning and strategies into the actual establishment of programs and product lines takes financial resources. The AHC cannot print money. Thus, one of three things must first happen: 1) increased revenues; 2) decreased expenses; or 3) a combination of the first two.

Within that context of the need for financial resources, the Chairs need to recognize the very positive economic engine that a robust AHC can be for a city or region. This role for the AHC as a vital economic-growth industry and as a major employer puts great pressure on the leaders of the AHC—the Senior Leaders and the Department Chairs. These Chairs have their essential roles: a) to ensure economic vitality and product service line development (see chapter 5); and b) to help in the creation of intellectual property, resulting in start-up companies in the region (see chapters 30 and 32).

Thus, the middle leaders in research, in clinical affairs, and in educational efforts are mandated to find resources—and yet at the same time charged with the task of being idealistic, generous, and giving. How can one best balance hard economic realities with the ideals of the medical profession—be those of the MD, the MD/PhD, the PhD, the nurses, the physician assistant, or the other staff?

> *"When you walk through a storm, hold your head up high, and don't be afraid of the dark.... Walk on, walk on through the wind and the rain.... At the end of the storm is a golden sky and the sweet silver song of the lark."*
>
> —FROM RICHARD RODGERS AND OSCAR HAMMERSTEIN II
> (FROM THE MUSICAL *CAROUSEL!*)

There are several superb, erudite dissertations on professionalism (3, 4, 5, 8, 10, 11, 25, 26, 30, 37, 42, and 43). All deal with the attributes of a profession, how to distinguish a profession from a discipline, and what makes a profession different from a commercial endeavor.

What makes a profession, as exemplified by the physician-patient relationship, the nurse-patient relationship, the physician-nurse interaction, the MD-PhD collaboration, and the Chair-faculty relationship, different from the relationship between a provider and a consumer?

There are five key features of a profession that these scholars define.

1) A profession engages in a societal or social service—it has altruism.

Professions must provide services above and beyond the necessary minimum because of an underlying service motive that transcends the desire for monetary gain. AHCs are entering an era where constricting resources and reimbursements for clinical care, research funding, and educational support threaten to destroy any sense of altruism—doing the right thing for the right reasons. Dr. Jordan Cohen, a past President of the AAMC in his article in the *Chicago Tribune*, said it clearly and with force: "The current market-oriented, cost-obsessed health-care system is intruding into the sanctity of the examining room.... Unlike typical transactions in the commercial marketplace, where suspicion is the watch cry, encounters with doctors cannot meet people's basic need without an atmosphere of trust. When ill, patients must have complete confidence that their doctor will act in their interest." (5) Against these forces, the Chair must espouse altruistic professionalism and ideals, and at the same time avoid the Mary Poppins Syndrome of unfounded optimism, by marshaling facts to support his/her position and thus lead by example.

2) A profession has the requirement for special education, training, and a high degree of knowledge.

A profession provides essential intellectual services, which require mastery of a substantial body of specialized knowledge, knowledge that is more than ordinarily complex.

3) Those within a profession have the ability and willingness to apply this knowledge and skill to a greater societal good.

A profession participates actively in a strong voluntary organization dedicated to the advancement and improvement in the type of services rendered. A profession applies theoretical and complex knowledge to the practical solution of human and societal problems. A profession strives to add to and improve its store of knowledge. Thus, professionals have a commitment to advance knowledge within their area of interest and expertise. Professionals in the healing arts must educate and pass the knowledge of the healing arts, medical research, and education on to the next generation. AHCs are threatened by financial collapse due to evolving governmental and insurance actions, which are threatening the professional mission.

4) A profession has autonomy—that is, the right to self-regulate.

A profession offers services in specialized areas that the general public is not trained in and is therefore unable to appraise or evaluate in terms of quality. A profession should therefore be free from uninhibited and irresponsible competition, and thus be able to foster education, patient care, and research in an atmosphere of dignity and self-respect. A profession is recognized by peers who may evaluate the quality of services rendered, based on factors more important than financial success. These evaluating and regulating bodies include the National Institutes of Health (NIH) with policies and study sections assessing research merit and financial support. For the areas of clinical care and clinical education these professional standards come from such as the Joint Commission for the Accreditation of Healthcare Organizations (JCAHO), the Liason Committee on Medical Education (LCME), the Accreditation Council for Graduate Medical Education (ACGME), the Residency Review Committees (RRCs), the American Board of Medical

Specialties (ABMS), and other such organizations. These professional systems establish rigorous criteria for research, for education, for clinical care and for proper conduct. Yet the ill-informed public and press judge the quality of care by the ambiance of the waiting room or the number of stitches in the skin. Similarly from lack of knowledge, the public and the press mock research on such things as yeast or the zebra fish, not appreciating the vast implications basic discoveries will have in advancing human health.

5) Conformance to and development of a body of ethics.

A profession observes a code of ethical conduct and communicates to the general public the professional standards the public has the right to expect.

Thus, there are five key attributes to a profession:

- Altruism

- Specialized education, leading to a high degree of knowledge

- Application of that education and knowledge to the greater good of society

- Autonomy to self-regulate

- Ethical standards

> *"Be more concerned with your character than your reputation, because your character is what you really are, while your reputation is merely what others think you are."*
>
> —JOHN WOODEN

Addressing the clinical area of effort nationally, McCullough states: "The essence of professionalism in medicine is the willingness of the physician to value the patient's welfare above his or her own. It is unselfish attention to the welfare of others and advocacy for our patients that earns the public's respect and trust." (25)

. . . .

Be a Leader
Make a Difference
Enjoy!

. . . .

21

Variations in the Organization and Disorganization of the AHC: Common Threads to Help the New Chair

"We tend to meet any new situation by reorganizing...and [what] a wonderful method it can be for creating the illusion of progress while producing inefficiency and demoralization."

—PETRONIUS

CHAPTER 4

The Unique Complexities of the AHC and the Resultant Implications for Leadership by Chairs

> *"Life isn't about waiting for the storm to pass. It's about learning to dance in the rain."*
> —VIVIAN GREENE

> *"How few there are who have courage enough to own their faults, or resolution enough to mend them."*
> —BENJAMIN FRANKLIN

1) **Key Points for the Chair to consider on AHC structure and function:**

   a) There is no single uniform table of organization. Great variations exist in different AHCs.

      i) Some AHCs own a hospital, some several hospitals, and some no hospital.

      ii) Some AHCs have clinic buildings within the AHC; others have them at a distance. Some AHCs own these off-site buildings, and others have established some variant of lease arrangements.

iii) Some AHCs have satellites; others do not. These satellites may be regional within a few hundred miles or less; some AHCs have satellites thousands of miles away in other states.

iv) Some AHCs have their own free-standing outpatient surgical centers. Other AHCs use external for-profit surgi-centers.

v) Some AHCs have a single CEO to whom the Dean, hospital(s), and all other Senior Leaders report. Other AHCs have very different reporting relationships, often driven by the presence or absence of a University connection and by the presence or absence of hospital ownership. Therefore, some AHCs have multiple "equal" leaders, which may include some or all of the deans, hospital directors, and one or several chief financial officers.

vi) As a result, some AHCs have rigid, centralized top-down control, whereas others are much more decentralized.

vii) Some AHCs have one or more competing AHCs in the same city; others are the "only gorilla in town."

viii) Some AHCs have as many as thirty-five to forty different Departments. Other AHCs have combined disciplines into larger Departments, reducing the overall number of Departments (such as having divisions of ENT, Plastic, Neurosurgery all part of the Department of Surgery, or combining Physiology and Pharmacology in one Department, and Biochemistry and Biophysics into another).

ix) Some AHCs are heavily weighted on the side of research with much more modest clinical activity, whereas others focus on robust clinical deliverables but with limited research.

x) Some have robust basic science research within clinical Departments. Some do not permit this, and all basic science is done within traditional basic science Departments.

xi) Some AHCs have a rigid "silo mentality" with little collaboration between Departments, and in fact may have competition such that "your enemy is across the hall and your best friend is down the street." Other AHCs have made real efforts to form bridges of collaboration among Departments to form research centers and/or clinical programs.

xii) Some AHCs have clinical faculty revenues mixed with hospital assets. Other AHCs have separate accounts for clinical faculty income, and these may be individual-based or Department-based, or may combine the incomes from all clinical Departments.

xiii) **Thus, "when a Chair has seen one AHC, he/she has seen one AHC."** The successful Chair will need the perception and wisdom to discern the nuggets of core issues, prudent goals and strategies, and be cognizant of those who might share his/her visions.

> *"An expert is a man who tells you a simple thing in a confused way in such a fashion as to make you think the confusion is your own fault."*
> —WILLIAM CASTLE, MD, HARVARD PROFESSOR OF MEDICINE
> (1924—68)

b) Not only are AHCs varied in the organizational structure that is selected and utilized, but great complexity also exists within whatever organizational structure is in place for that particular AHC. Thus, a Chair seeking one-size-fits-all leadership will be confounded by complexity compounded by complexity. The reasons for these organizational variations are dictated by: 1) the multiple varied missions, often influenced by local and regional factors; 2) powerful external economic, political, and public forces (see chapter 5); and c) the incredibly complex breadth and depth of "product lines" of the AHC.

c) These "product lines" are for the benefit of today's and tomorrow's patients via research, education, patient care, and community outreach. *But*, "no money, no mission," and hence, the mission idealism must confront and accept the realities of the essential needs for business plans, legal issues, compliance regulations, intellectual property and technology transfer, and external inspecting and credentialing bodies.

> *"Courage and perseverance have a magic talisman before which difficulties disappear and obstacles vanish into thin air."*
>
> —JOHN QUINCY ADAMS

d) Only the MDs, the PhDs, the MD/PhDs, the DOs, DPhils, PsyDs, and those with other doctoral degrees will have the skill, knowledge, vision, and ability to identify key current product lines in their highly subspecialized, complex, and sophisticated scientific area(s) of expertise. Only these doctoral leaders will have the expertise and the vision to create, implement, and drive successful new product lines. But these MDs and PhDs and MD/PhDs will be doomed to failure if they rely solely on their own abilities.

   i) The MDs and PhDs need a tight linkage to MBAs and legal experts for the development of sound business and legal basis for products. There is the need to tighten the cross-linkages between these skill sets by: a) having more MDs and PhDs with second degrees in business/law; or b) having the MDs and PhDs work closely in partnership with those who have those skill sets (the author favors "b," as "a" often creates the downfall for the Chair who is knowledgeable in many areas but expert in none).

ii) Problems are, and will become much more, challenging from increasing external pressures from NIH, Medicare, Medicaid, the insurance industry, states and municipalities, and the federal government.

iii) Thus, the individual Chair has an essential leadership role to fulfill, and there are aspects under his/her control.

2) The Chairs have a prime role in "product line" conception, creation, organization, and delivery. Only the Chairs (or Center Directors) will have the expertise to know what new creative opportunities exist in their sphere of medical expertise to possibly become "hot," "key," "promising." Examples of product lines are limitless: a stream of well-educated resident trainees, licensing agreements/patents for new vaccines for cancer, new PhD programs, or coordinated care across Departments for cardiac disease, etc. Regardless of whatever organizational format is in place or is contemplated, at the *hub of activity there are Chairs*, each responsible for his/her discipline(s), and responsible for delivering a "product"—or usually several "products." It is key to remember that these products, regardless of type, are *for the benefit of patients—be it immediate or in the more distant future, be it for the single patient(s) or for a population.* And often these products involve several of areas simultaneously and to varying extents:

a) Education—medical students, residents, fellows, and/or MS/PhD graduate students

b) Research—extensive or limited, basic science, clinical studies, and/or translational research

c) Patient care—delivered by physicians with or without nurse practitioners and/or physician assistants

d) Community outreach—population health, outreach clinics, and/ or educational programs in regional high schools

e) Fiscal responsibility—clinical revenue (billed centrally or by Department) and/or research revenues (with or without indirect reimbursements). Ideally the Chair is responsible for revenues and has the authority to make fiscal decisions; although, again this varies tremendously from one AHC to another

3) These product line initiatives as proposed and possibly implemented by a Chair, or ideally by several Chairs working in concert, must fit within and enhance the mission statement and visions espoused by the Senior Leadership of the AHC. These Chair efforts also need to recognize the task to adjust to changing institutional priorities and leadership in response to evolving challenges, while at the same time the Chair works to maintain (and even enhance) faculty morale.

"It always seems impossible until it's done."
—NELSON MANDELA

4) As shown above, it is apparent that there are many variables, but there are also some constants:

a) The Chair will have essential and varied relationships:

i) With those to whom he/she reports (Dean or Deans, one or more Chief Financial Officers, perhaps indirectly or directly to a CEO)

ii) With peers at the "same level" (other Chairs)—some from larger units, some from smaller units, and hence there may be tiers of peers—especially for multi-Departmental disease-focused programs

iii) With faculty who report to the Chair

iv) With staff who are responsible to the Chair

b) The successes and failures of AHCs, and the successes and failures of Departments within an AHC, are often varied and uneven. There are several pivotal factors:

i) The leadership provided by Senior Leadership

ii) The leadership of the Chair or Chairs involved; in multi-Departmental efforts, the leadership skills, or lack thereof, in one Department contrasted with another are important to consider

iii) Patient and population needs

iv) Finances and other resources—both internal and external to the AHC

v) Governmental and other external funding agency perceptions of "what is important to fund" (research, clinical care, and/or education)

c) The most successful AHC, to a large degree, can look to multiple, successful Departments working collaboratively as "the guts" of the successful larger AHC organization.

d) The Chairs and leaders of Centers and Programs propel "the guts" of the AHC, and thus *lead from the middle* (see chapter 5).

. . . .

Be a Leader
Make a Difference
Enjoy!

. . . .

CHAPTER 5

. . . .

The Chair's Essential Role in Middle Leadership is *Not* an Oxymoron in the Robust AHC

> *"A lot can be accomplished if you don't care who gets the credit."*
>
> —KENNETH G. BURTON, MD, TO HIS SON, RICHARD, 1958

1) "Middle leadership" should be considered first class, not second class. Chairs function as "middle leadership," as they report to those above, and are responsible for resources, faculty, staff, and deliverables. As detailed in the prior chapter, Chairs are the engines that generate the new and productive ideas for new product lines, new research opportunities, and new educational tools. Several aspects of this merit comment:

   a) Great CEOs and great Deans are critically important, but without effective Chair leadership, the AHC is much less able to thrive in its multiple missions.

   b) In clinical Departments, only the MD, MD/PhD, DO, and PsyD have the skill sets and the knowledge to deal successfully with opportunities and challenges imposed by RRCs and the ACGME, by changes in NIH regulations and funding lines, by possible productive product lines, and by "lost leaders" in clinical care.

   c) In both clinical and basic science disciplines, the enormous explosion of knowledge demands sub-sub-specialized expertise and, by implication, thereby increases the need for collaborations among Departments and disciplines.

d) Great Chairs are critically important, but without effective creative and visionary leadership by the Senior Leaders, these Chairs cannot produce "good products." There is an enormous need for institutional vision, mission, clarity, and creativity rooted in the team concept.

2) Chairs truly need to relate effectively in three directions—a) with those to whom they report (Senior Leadership); b) with those who report to them (Departmental faculty and staff); and c) with those at their level (other Chairs). Superb "middle leadership" by Chairs is essential for successes of the AHC, especially long-term successes.

   a) Neither brick-and-mortar nor business and legal personnel do research, see patients, do surgeries, or have clinical and/or research expertise.

   b) Yet both business and legal expertise and appropriate physical facilities are essential to deliver the product line(s) for patient benefits, now and in the future.

      i) Physical resources are essential to house, equip, and make possible the product line creation and delivery.

      ii) Both business and legal expertise are essential for the MDs, MD/PhDs, and PhDs to create: a) sound business plans; and b) legal structures and strategies. With the ever-increasing financial and legal complexities of the external environment, failure to assimilate such business and legal expertise into the visionary and practical planning by the AHC can be catastrophic.

3) Chairs must collaborate with each other within the AHC and with Senior Leadership during strategic planning, to develop multi-Departmental efforts in clinical service lines, in research, and in

educational programs. In fact there are strong, prudent reasons for research Chairs and for clinical Chairs to develop strong collaborations between AHCs as well as within their own AHC to facilitate the creative growth of "big science" from cross-disciplinary and cross-institutional research efforts and studies.

4) Production Programs will involve any combination of patient care, education (MD, PhD, residents, fellows, continuing medical education), and research (basic science, clinical, translational)—all necessary for, and justified by, the care of today's and tomorrow's patients. The Chairs are essential with key roles, yet with major challenges to conceive, create, and deliver. As mentioned previously, *product lines* is a term used to indicate the result of focused AHC effort and resources with the strategic goal to significantly improve the care of patients and populations today and in the future by coordinated educational, research, and clinical commitments. Examples of product lines might include:

   a) Neural Medicine: this would include Neurology, Neurosurgery, Neural Imaging, and all clinical and basic Neurosciences

   b) Musculoskeletal: this would include Orthopaedics (Spine, Adult Reconstruction, Pediatric Orthopaedics, Foot/Ankle, Shoulder/Elbow, Hand, Musculoskeletal Oncology, Sports Medicine, Trauma, Microsurgery, and Replantation), Musculoskeletal research, Rehabilitation, Rheumatology, Musculoskeletal Imaging

   c) Cardiovascular: this would include Cardiology, Cardiac Surgery, Vascular diseases, Vascular Surgery, Cardiovascular Imaging, and research in all these areas

   d) Cancer—medical, surgical, and research aspects

   e) Educational teaching products—multidisciplinary revenue-generating programs such as new certificate programs or masters programs (ideally using largely extant resources and courses, thus avoiding the need for incremental resources)

> *"Even if you are on the right track, you will get run over if you just sit there."*
> —WILL ROGERS

5) Problems and challenges in creating and delivering product lines have origins that are both external and internal to the AHC and include, but certainly are not limited to:

   a) External:

      i) ACGME/RRC issues, with this as an example: Imaging Sciences and Anesthesiology are essential to and part of each product line—how can the AHC maintain educational and training integrity of these two nationally recognized and nationally regulated disciplines, so as to enhance the product line and yet still satisfy RRC and ACGME requirements in those specialties?

      ii) Social services

      iii) Patient transport, such as surface and air ambulance services

      iv) Third-party carriers who will need some sort of billing and accounting systems unique to the AHC, as these coordinated multi-discipline products usually are not provided and not realistic at other types of health-care facilities

      v) Compliance with and avoidance of Stark Law issues

   b) The intertwining roles of multiple Departments in multiple product lines, results in any single Department being involved in multiple product lines, but each of the separate product lines having a different constellation of involved Departments.

This leads to very complex challenges for resource allocation, expense allocation, and revenue distribution. As one example of the types of program product lines, consider transplantation of solid organs and transplantation of limbs. All involve the primary care networks, which both are the source of the patients and must be coordinated into the follow-up care, making these patients far more complex and time-consuming than many other patients for primary care personnel. Examples of multi-specialty involvement in various combinations needed for transplantation include:

i) Kidney—involves Medicine (Nephrology, Infectious Disease), Immunology (both clinical and research), Pediatrics on occasion, Urology and/or Surgery, Anesthesia, Imaging Sciences

ii) Liver—involves Medicine (GI, Infectious Disease), Pediatrics upon occasion, Immunology (both clinical and research), Surgery, Anesthesia, Imaging Sciences, intensive care expertise

iii) Lung—involves Medicine (Pulmonary, Infectious Disease), Pediatrics upon occasion, Immunology (clinical and basic science), Thoracic Surgery, Anesthesia, Imaging Sciences, intensive care expertise

iv) Heart—involves Surgery, Cardiac Surgery, Medicine (Cardiology, Infectious Disease), Pediatrics on occasion, Immunology (both clinical and basic science), Anesthesia, Imaging Sciences, intensive care expertise

v) Limb—involves Orthopaedics, Immunology (both clinical and research), Psychiatry

c) All of these product lines are necessary for optimal care, are expensive even with all efforts to streamline and standardize, and are a disadvantage to the AHC's "efficiency" and its ability to compete for cost with standard community hospitals.

d) Within the AHC as these product lines mature, they will continually change with new scientific advances. Very importantly, these product lines will also change with patient demographics, such as the aging population, the emergence of new diseases such as AIDS, the disappearance of diseases such as polio, and the declining incidence of diseases such as cerebral palsy.

e) The business organizational demands will be real. There will be significant internal resource, expense, and revenue allocations. Coordination of billing services and compliance regulations, as well as development of equitable and competitive faculty salary structures, will be challenging.

f) These multi-Departmental efforts, building collaborative bridges and not fences between Departments and Programs, result in research, clinical efforts, and teaching across traditional Departmental lines. This results in the need for modification of AHC administration and policies. Examples include the tracking of clinical revenues to responsible Departments and the resultant multiple PIs on single research grants imposing the need to modify promotion requirements, especially for tenure. (see Appendices B, C, and D.)

6) Only the Chairs of the involved Departments will have the necessary medical knowledge base of current medical sciences and treatments and, very importantly, a sense of where the real opportunities will be in the future for new products needed by the populations being served. *Very importantly*, these Chairs and leaders *must* be able to (and here is a real challenge):

a) Develop strong and sincere collaborations with Chairs of the other involved Departments

b) For his/her Department, infuse that collaborative spirit into the other faculty, the involved nursing services, the residents and fellows, and the associated staff at all levels

c) Work with Senior Leadership and the other Chairs to identify realistic multi-Departmental innovative programs to target clinical and research opportunities

d) Work with Senior Leadership and other Chairs to prioritize and establish timelines for these new multi-Departmental efforts

e) Work with Senior Leadership and other Chairs to create for the preceding programs the necessary project-specific budgets of space, time, and money that are mission-focused and fair to each and every one of the involved Departments

Be a Leader
Make a Difference
Enjoy!

38

SECTION III

The Partnership of the AHC and the Faculty for Leadership Development

"To each there comes in their lifetime a special moment when they are figuratively tapped on the shoulder and offered the chance to do a very special thing, unique to them and fitted to their talents. What a tragedy if that moment finds them unprepared or unqualified for that which could have been their finest hour."

—WINSTON CHURCHILL

"The value of an education...is not the learning of many facts, but the training of the mind to think of something that cannot be learned from textbooks."

—ALBERT EINSTEIN

> *"It is the business of the teacher to arouse curiosity, not to satisfy it. The measure of a teacher's success lies not in his [her] own ideas but in those which radiate from his [her] pupils."*
>
> —HARVEY CUSHING, MD, *CONSECRATIO MEDICI*

CHAPTER 6

. . . .

"Gestational Stages of Leaders In Utero"

"Every path has a few puddles."
—ORIGINAL AUTHOR UNKNOWN

Both the AHC and the aspiring faculty have obligations in leadership development. The AHCs have the opportunity and responsibility to develop and nurture emerging faculty of notable promise, grooming them for eventual leadership positions in that same AHC or another one (see chapter 7). These young, talented faculty also have obligations in this process (see chapter 8).

There are career phases where young and midcareer faculty have opportunities to enhance their reputation as reliable, creative, productive, mature contributors who collaborate well, are team players, and yet are independent thinkers with emerging potential to be leaders.

What should a faculty member do proactively to position him/herself to develop a career where he/she could be considered as a Chair candidate either within his/her institution or at another AHC?

Regarding this relationship with the emerging leaders within an AHC, the philosophy should be one of win-win. The emerging leader wins because new talents are recognized and skills are developed that position that younger person for future leadership at that AHC or as a candidate for such leadership at another AHC. The AHC wins in two ways: 1) within the AHC new leaders emerge, positioned for greater leadership responsibility to move the AHC forward; and b) rather than training new leaders who might go elsewhere, paradoxically these new emerging leaders see the host AHC as nurturing and mentoring and interested in his/her career advancement, and therefore do not see the need to leave for another AHC to continue the upward career trajectory. This desired trajectory can occur in the host AHC.

The AHC, in broad terms, can consider faculty in one of three phases—to draw an analogy from Obstetrics—the first trimester, the second trimester, and the third trimester. The structure and purpose of the mentoring is progressive and different in each trimester. The duration of time spent by each faculty member in each trimester, unlike in fetal development, is not determined by the calendar but rather by the abilities of the faculty member, the nature of the career, and various personal matters such as family responsibilities or health issues. Furthermore, the passage from one career trimester to the next can be a blurred timeline and often is not a sudden "click" from one phase to the next. In each of these trimesters, the faculty member as mentee has significant matching responsibilities; these are detailed in Chapter 8.

> *"The best sermons are lived, not preached."*
> —ORIGINAL AUTHOR UNKNOWN

1) The first trimester of faculty leadership development is one of formation, of differentiation. Training in clinical, educational, and/or research disciplines is merely the launch pad; the early faculty years are the launch of the career. In most AHCs, these faculty will be Senior Instructors and/or Assistant Professors. In most situations the final career trajectory may not be obvious early on. Will this faculty member emerge as a great researcher, a great clinician, a great educator, or a combination of these? What innate potential skills and talents need to be recognized by the individual faculty and the AHC? One-on-one mentoring is important, and the mentor may need to change if the major potential strengths are different from first predicted. In addition to the one-on-one mentoring, group

mentoring by senior faculty is essential. Such group topics include organizational tables of the AHC; how to develop teaching skills and educational scholarship; how to mature as a clinician with a focused area of expertise; how to successfully write grants to obtain extramural funding; what is involved in administering a successful research lab; issues related to conflicts of interest, compliance, and institutional review boards; development of a résumé biography and curriculum vitae; and navigating the promotion system.

2) In the second trimester, once career-path differentiation has occurred into the descriptors of researcher-teacher, researcher-teacher-clinician, clinician-teacher, or scholarly teacher-clinician, the AHC mentoring takes on two new additional efforts: 1) fostering the emergence of faculty onto the national stage with reputation in research, clinical care, and/or education prowess; and 2) fostering their advancement into early leadership roles within the AHC. Some of these faculty academic appointments will be in the last year as Assistant Professor, and for many others at the rank of Associate Professor.

   a) How can the AHC foster the national profile? The early emergence will require success from the first trimester, with funded NIH research and/or substantive publications. In the latter portions of the first trimester and especially in the early second trimester, the mentor needs to push national connections for the mentee. For example, the mentor can decline a position on a national panel or decline to be a visiting professor, saying to the inviter, "Normally I'd be honored to do this, but my commitments preclude this. However, I have a younger colleague who is fantastic with similar expertise. He/she would be great for this. Here's how to reach her/him." Also, in this trimester, the mentor needs to not place his/her name on papers of the mentee, in order to establish the intellectual independence of the mentee.

   b) The fostering of leadership development within the AHC means many obligations for the AHC "system" and the mentor. The

AHC needs to have a formal leadership educational program within the institution, or send the faculty member to one of the several nationally given programs. The curriculum for such programs needs to cover most of the topics in this book. One-on-one the mentor and mentee need to identify and capitalize on committee openings and opportunities within the institution that allow the faculty member to productively participate—be that on credentialing committees, compliance committees, review committees, thesis committees, admission committees, etc.

> *"Treat a man [woman] as if he [she] were what he [she] ought to be and you help him [her] become what he [she] is capable of being."*
> —JOHANN VON GOETHE

3) By the third trimester, these faculty will have professorial academic appointments and now serve as mentors to younger faculty. The established faculty member will him/herself soon be a serious candidate for a major AHC leadership position, such as Departmental Chair, and will often already be the head of a Division within a large Department, lead major committees within the AHC, have a significant national presence in major organizations, and/or, if in research, will sit on an NIH study section. These leadership and administrative roles will give these faculty members a track record of substance, making the individual a legitimate candidate for a Chair position.

. . . .

Be a Leader
Make a Difference
Enjoy!

. . . .

CHAPTER 7

Pros and Cons of AHCs "Growing Their Own" Leaders

> *"If you see a turtle on a fence post, you'll know it never got there by itself."*
>
> —FRANK WILSON, MD

There are many cogent reasons for AHCs to have established mentoring and leadership development programs in place. They are powerful ways to optimize the organizational efficiency and productivity of the AHC. Such programs can provide a strong, positive stimulus for faculty satisfaction and retention (see chapter 6).

What assets should the AHC commit to such programs? These assets include the cost of time and the cost of meeting space, even if no external consultants or programs are involved. The net cost of time is hard to quantify. Any hours spent by the mentors and mentees are hours not spent generating clinical revenues, not spent doing research, and not spent writing grants. But these costs need to be netted out against subsequent increases in productivity across the AHC. This productivity will be the result of more success in grant funding by younger faculty and/or by more vibrant and successful clinical programs. Very importantly, significant increases in productivity across the AHC will be the result of stronger internal leadership skills subsequently exhibited by faculty who've benefited from leadership development. The one-on-one mentoring does not involve space, but the formal leadership topical sessions will. Because of busy faculty hours, such space is usually needed early in the morning, late in the day, or on weekends, and hence, teaching facilities will usually be available at no significant extra cost.

Hopefully from such leadership programs, very strong internal candidates will emerge for Chair searches, be these searches in basic science or clinical Departments. That said, from the perspectives of the AHC and of the candidates, what is the role of the internal candidate in such searches? What are the relative advantages and disadvantages of internal vs. external candidate appointments to Chair positions after a search?

The proper role for an internal candidate should be as a legitimate leader, a viable candidate for the Chair position. The internal candidate should not be a "token." If the AHC has had a solid leadership development program, there should emerge at least one strong internal candidate for the Chair position. This individual should have the stature to be a viable Chair candidate at another AHC if he/she so decided. The internal candidate should be selected only as part of a national search, for to do so will augment the credibility, credentials, and value of the internal candidate as the next Chair (see chapter 10).

> *"Dig the well before you are thirsty."*
> —Chinese Proverb

From the perspective of the Senior Leadership of the AHC, the internal candidate has advantages.

1) The internal candidate will be well-known, and the Senior Leadership should have a strong sense of the internal candidate's strengths and weaknesses. But the "known warts" will be in the candidate's prior role or roles. The skill sets needed by the Chair may exceed the internal candidate's prior experiences, and he/she may exhibit problems previously not known.

> *"Never buy a car you can't push."*
> —Author unknown

2) The successful, very strong internal candidate speaks to the excellence of the AHC's leadership development programs, and reaffirms the outstanding caliber of that Department's faculty.

3) The internal candidate should not be viewed by Senior Leadership as the "cheapest" to recruit, so ideally the internal candidacy should not be an economic advantage to the AHC (unfortunately not always the case). That said, Senior Leadership will have a more solid sense of the value of this candidate as a potential new leader, especially if the AHC has a viable leadership development program. If this person were at another AHC and being recruited as Chair, would this individual be of such merit that Senior Leadership would invest major resources in the recruitment package, and how much would that be, knowing what they do about this internal candidate? This can be a very valid perspective for Senior Leadership to consider as they evaluate the internal candidate as the best candidate.

4) The internal candidate knows the AHC and knows "the cast of characters." This will provide the opportunity for the internal candidate to focus on the major areas for improvement in the Department, with a much more insightful strength-weakness-opportunity-threat (SWOT) analysis.

5) The internal leader is better positioned to negotiate realistically for essential items, as he/she should have a solid sense of what is truly needed to move the Department forward.

As viewed by Senior Leadership what advantages does the external candidate possess, and what are the risks inherent in the external candidate?

1) The external candidate in theory will bring in fresh ideas and new insights for what the Department needs in order to flourish.

2) If the external candidate is a major national figure, he/she may enhance the reputation of the AHC.

3) The Department faculty may feel positively about getting the strong external candidate because they believe that this speaks to their own excellence (they are so good they attracted the high-profile external person).

4) The external candidate may be able to bring with him/her other outstanding faculty from the prior AHC.

5) The external candidate may well want to negotiate for a richer recruitment package.

6) The external candidate, even with the best of due diligence, is a relative unknown. He/she may have major flaws, unrecognized and not apparent with due-diligence efforts. It can be hugely expensive for the AHC if the new Chair has to be dismissed.

7) The external candidate will not know the intricacies and histories of the AHC, and hence will have a more difficult and longer learning curve.

Thus, an excellent case can be made for an imaginative, vibrant, and well-executed leadership development program that positions the AHC to have such solid internal Chair candidates as to position the AHC to select very strong internal candidates after a national search. "The best candidate is right here and is well-known to us."

Be a Leader
Make a Difference
Enjoy!

CHAPTER 8

Each Faculty Member Has the Challenge and Responsibility to Emerge as a Potential Leader

> *"Hard work pays off in the future.*
> *Laziness pays off now."*
> —AUTHOR UNKNOWN

> *"I will prepare and some day my chance will come."*
> —ABRAHAM LINCOLN

Just as the AHC has opportunities and responsibilities to nurture and develop future academic leaders, the faculty at AHC who aspire to career advancement with more leadership opportunities have the obligation to show interest, availability, and effort on their own behalf. This is true in all "three trimesters of faculty gestational age" (see chapter 6). The individual faculty member needs to take personal ownership of enhancing his/her skills, roles, and responsibilities within his/her Department, the AHC, and nationally—and to do so without being inappropriately "pushy," aggressive, and self-serving. Each of these promising early- and midcareer faculty must recognize that in being nurtured, he/she is being watched and assessed for performance, potential, and style. How much does each of these emerging faculty leaders demonstrate "fire in the belly, but with grace" vs. "fire in the belly with elbows out, trampling all in his/her path"? How much does each of these emerging faculty show a capacity for hard work as a productive team player with vision vs. the hard worker who labors only as a follower, not a leader?

Demonstrating loyalty to their own AHC is important for emerging leaders. They must be active participants in the leadership development programs of the AHC—an active learner, not someone who says, "I'll sit back and be spoon-fed because the AHC owes me this." Just as outlined in Chapter 6 that paradoxically the fostering of leadership development in younger faculty enhances their desire to remain at the host AHC, so the paradox exists that by demonstrating firm allegiance to the host AHC, the emerging leader maximally enhances his/her reputation as a reliable, trustworthy potential star and thus becomes more attractive for recruiting by another AHC. Thus the firm mutual commitment between the AHC and that AHC's "leaders in training" is a true win-win.

> *"I've learned that you can tell a lot about a person by the way he/she handles these three things: a rainy day, lost luggage, and tangled Christmas tree lights."*
> —MAYA ANGELOU

The three phases of faculty development are detailed in Chapter 6, the role of the AHC in Chapter 7, and in summary, here is what the AHC expects from the emerging faculty member leader.

1) For the young faculty member in the first trimester who might be aspiring to some future leadership position, the groundwork for this is initiated early on. The first step is for him/her to look inward for personal thoughts on career goals and, based upon that, to seek out a mentor, a fellow faculty member well along on the career path that the young faculty member envisions as a possible trajectory for him/herself. If this more senior faculty member has not already initiated a mentor-mentee connection with the young faculty member, the latter should reach out to the possible mentor. Each needs to be

optimistic about the mentor-mentee arrangement, and should the career paths of either diverge, a new mentor should be sought. The mentor should encourage the young faculty member to avail him/herself to all the leadership development meetings or seminars available within the AHC, as referenced in the prior chapter. The one-on-one mentoring is very important and should be tailored to the unique situation of each young faculty member. The young faculty member may not know what he/she wants and may not recognize his/her own strengths. The firm, guiding "push" from the senior mentor for the mentee to take on some new responsibility can be of great help in the mentee's development and career trajectory. Give-and-take dialogues should range on many topics, with the older faculty member listening, encouraging, and sharing insights and personal experiences with lessons learned by the mentor in the course of his/her career. The mentee should be comfortable asking questions and seeking advice from the mentor. The mentee should not manufacture superficial nuisance questions, but rather seek guidance on well-thought-out alternative situational courses of action. The mentor will not only have the wisdom to guide in a positive sense but will also have the confidence to understand that "one of my responsibilities is to help you avoid all the mistakes I made along the way." Thus, the mentee needs to be just as active a participant in the mentor-mentee relationship as the mentor. Also, at this time the mentor should nurture in the mentee the attributes of being well-grounded, a team player, polite, honest, energetic, hardworking, creative, reliable, and enthusiastic. The mentee should seek out criticism—"How did I do with this? Any suggestions on how to do it better?" At this stage, it is key that the mentee complete any task or assignment given to him/her, delivering the requested report or assignment result on time. The mentee, if not already so accomplished, must be schooled on the delivering of both verbal and written reports. Even though understandably nervous, the mentee should be coached by the mentor on how to deliver a committee report thoughtfully, clearly, concisely, in a measured pace, with handouts if indicated, and to be ready to answer factually any questions or challenges that might arise. Toward the end of the first trimester, as soon as the mentor deems the mentee ready, the mentor should push senior leadership to appoint the mentee to more influential committees within the AHC—both for the experience involved, but also to facilitate the mentee's contacts across many other Departments and/or areas of the AHC. In the course of this latter part of the first trimester, the mentee should be certain that the mentor is aware that he/she is very willing to substitute for the mentor in local, regional, or national events and assignments should the mentor's calendar preclude him/her from doing this.

2) The second trimester for the mentee will often blend into the first trimester without a sharp demarcation. The mentee, with the successful increase in responsibility at the AHC, will have carefully observed what does and does not seem to be effective behavior by various Chairs, Center Directors, and other AHC leaders. The mentee will have successfully completed various committee responsibilities and will have attended leadership seminars within the AHC, seminars targeted at the younger faculty. At this time the mentor may or may not be changed. If the younger faculty career trajectory has modified, a smooth transition to another mentor might be advantageous to all involved.

The mentor should now actively foster the emergence of a national profile for the mentee by such as suggesting the mentee's name for committee assignments in national professional organizations in which they both belong. This will provide an increasing national profile for the mentee and at the same time provide the mentee with valuable experience. Now the mentee has major responsibilities to: a) keep the mentor informed on events and emerging responsibilities and seek advice as prudent; b) be a productive member of the national-level committee. The mentee should actively participate in this new national-level involvement and opportunity, and not be passive or insecure. This will take some skill by the mentee. On the one hand, he/she is "the new kid on the block" and initially will need to be an astute observer of people, of situations, of interactions, and of national "politics." When speaking out in this setting, the mentee will need to draw upon experiences from analogous committee assignments previously held at his/her AHC. In this role the mentee should speak with facts and with calm confidence, but not arrogance. Furthermore, the mentee will learn what does and does not work in such settings by observing leaders from other AHCs on how to get involved in national committee tasks and deliverables for the benefit of the national organization. At this stage of the mentee's career, the increase in experiences on more senior committees in the AHC, and simultaneously in national responsibilities, will each foster the other in developing leadership skills and help the mentee in becoming politically astute.

3) The third trimester is the time that the faculty member will have emerged as a leader within the AHC, will have risen through the academic ranks to a professorial appointment, and will have major positions in committee leadership in national committees of academic organizations. By this time, the mentee will have evolved into a mentor for others. The emerging leader most likely will have significant roles in the AHC, such as Division leader in a large Department, appointment as an Associate Chair, and/or leadership positions on major AHC committees. If they have not already done so, these individuals should attend one or more of the nationally recognized leadership courses.

· ·

Be a Leader
Make a Difference
Enjoy!

· ·

The Search Process—the Dating, the Engagement, and the Prenuptial Agreement (Offer Letter)

CHAPTER 9

What the AHC and the Candidate Should Expect in the Courtship of the Search Process

> *"Talent hits a target no one else can hit.*
> *Genius hits a target no one else can see."*
>
> —ARTHUR SCHOPENHAUER

The integrity, efficiency, and results of the many searches for academic Chairs in the AHC to a large measure will determine the future capabilities and quality of the AHC. How these searches are conducted varies from one AHC to another, and the results are uneven, regardless of the specifics of how the search is conducted.

The Senior Leadership of any AHC, as the result of an honest self-assessment, will have to attest to the uneven quality of Chairs, some excellent, some average, and some poor. This variation in Chair quality does not relate to whether that Chair came forward as an external or internal candidate, nor does it correlate with the "traditional" search process or with the use of a professional search firm.

Similarly, any current Chair of an academic Department in an AHC will admit to surprises, challenges, and frustrations in the role of Chair. Some of this is inherent in the nature of the Chair position, and some is perhaps the result of the need for better communication during the search process. This should lead to a more prudent and broad-based offer letter both defining the Chair's anticipated role and responsibilities and delineating the AHC's resources to be committed in support of the new Chair's upcoming endeavors.

There is a definite need to improve search processes for Chairs and other leadership positions in AHCs. First, there should be a higher success rate for satisfaction by both the AHC and the new Chair/leader. Second, and equally important, somehow the search process needs to be less protracted, more predictable, and with better due diligence on the part of both the AHC and the candidate. At the present time, the slowness of search processes is not yielding appropriate due diligence; equally important, the slowness of the process often causes interim disruptions and inefficiencies in the Department and the AHC at large (especially for critical and/or big Departments).

Recognizing the need for a better search process, AHCs are seeking better ways to search for new Chairs and are modifying approaches. Some AHCs make incremental adjustments, others radical changes. Regardless of how the AHC conducts a search, the AHC will have much more experience in the search process than will the individual candidate, whether that candidate is exploring his/her first Chair position or has looked previously.

There is some advice for candidates seeking Chair opportunities:

1) Be certain that his/her CV and bio-sketch are current and consistent with the information on the present website of the candidate's current AHC.

2) Be very aware of impending opportunities at his/her current AHC:

   a) Is the Chair position at his/her current institution soon to be available, and if so is he/she the leading internal candidate?

   b) Is the Chair position at his/her current institution occupied by a young and successful Chair, such that no opportunity will be available in the foreseeable future?

3) Consider the pros and cons of "quietly looking" vs. making it known he/she is in the market for moving to a Chair position. The positives are fostering the reputation of being open and above board and of

having the strong national reputation to justify the candidacy. The negatives are creating the perception that the candidate is restless and is not a good citizen within the current AHC and/or is trying to leverage a potential new position to gain more resources at the current home institution.

4) The person considering whether or not to enter a Chair search needs to assess how well connected is he/she nationally, for the purposes of:

   a) Getting strong reference letters and supporting phone calls when the due-diligence processes start as the searching AHC initiates inquiries on the final candidates

   b) "Getting the word out" that he/she would like to be a Chair candidate, so that influential contacts will provide his/her name to inquiring AHCs that are starting a search

5) Considerations on how frequently to be a candidate include:

   a) The overly frequent candidate may lead to perception that he/she is 1) looking at everything indiscriminately without exercising judgment; or 2) is leveraging these candidacies so that he/she can enhance a retention package at the current AHC or, at the other extreme, is desperate to leave because of baggage accumulated.

   b) The established senior faculty member who rarely seeks Chair candidacy may create the perception that he/she 1) is very content where he/she is; 2) lacks real desire to be a Chair; or 3) is not very competitive for a Chair position.

   c) Frequent candidacies without selection will lead to perceptions that he/she 1) must not be very competitive in failing so often to be selected; 2) must be an impossible person with whom to negotiate; or 3) asks consistently for too rich a recruitment package.

6) In summary, the faculty person seeking to become a Chair needs:

   a) To be prudently selective in candidacy

   b) Have a strong national position and an excellent record at his/her current AHC

   c) To be astute in assessing the strengths and weaknesses and the threats and opportunities of the inviting institution

   d) If negotiating, to do so with astute knowledge of and firm insights into the inviting AHC

7) The candidacy done with style and sincerity, even if not selected, will:

   a) Be a valuable learning experience in search processes

   b) Enhance his/her national reputation and lead to other search invitations

   c) Educate the candidate on beneficial changes to be implemented at his/her current AHC

The AHCs have many variations in how searches are conducted and Chairs are selected. Most searches for Chairs of major Departments are national searches, and most of these will seek multiple viable external candidates. Most will also include one or two internal candidates. Some of these searches are done utilizing resources internal to the AHC; other AHCs will contract with an external search firm.

Regardless of how these searches are currently conducted, the process is lengthy. It is of interest that major large businesses and professional sports teams can conduct searches for leadership positions that are successful in a time frame often measured in weeks. Contrast that with AHC searches that often can consume a year. The time invested is not necessarily correlated with the level of success of the subsequent Chair's performance.

The common steps in most AHC search processes are methodical:

1) The current Chair vacates; the situation and reasons vary.

   a) Ideally this is a cordial event, with the Chair electing to step aside, and with the Dean's agreement and sincere regrets. In this desirable situation, hopefully the current Chair will agree to remain in place until the new Chair arrives. This will avoid what can be a very difficult transition with an interim or acting Chair.

   b) The most difficult scenario precipitating the need for a Chair search is the poor performance of the current Chair with a Department in decline. In these cases, the Dean, in essence, "fires" the Chair. Often, to save face, the Chair is offered the opportunity "to resign as Chair to pursue other interests." This may result in: 1) the Chair retiring and exiting the AHC; 2) the Chair remaining in the Department "to pursue his/her clinical and/or research interests"; or 3) the Chair moving to another Department or Center. The best for the Department is the first. The other two alternatives, especially the second, leave the departing Chair in a position to be very disruptive via those faculty who retain an allegiance to him/her.

2) Should the transition time between Chairs involve an acting or interim Chair, matters may become less stable in the Department. This temporary Chair is faced with the challenge of not just holding the Department together, but of hopefully even moving the Department forward if the search is prolonged. This is an exceedingly difficult task, because this temporary Chair has almost no traction, being perceived as a "lame duck." Faculty may think, "Why should I agree to do Z? Why should I follow? You won't be here long." Other Chairs may view the temporary Chair as a "short-termer," providing the other Chairs with little or no need or justification to collaborate with the interim leader. During a transition

time with an acting Chair, Senior Leadership can be exceedingly helpful in providing strong links to the Dean's Office and firm mentoring and backing for the interim Departmental leadership. Unfortunately, this is often not the situation, as Senior Leadership may understandably decide, "Why should the AHC give any resources to the interim situation? Let's wait to see what the new Chair will want, and save our resources for the new Chair negotiations." That may or may not be wise, as an interim period that is long in the absence of AHC support will weaken the Department, make it less attractive for a new Chair, and in the long run require a more lucrative recruitment package.

3) A search committee (SC) is appointed.

   a) This may occur immediately, or be delayed until after the Dean considers whether or not the Department will be retained, restructured, or combined with another Department.

   b) The Dean may select the SC independent of input, or the Dean may consult with other Senior Leadership as to the composition of the committee for various academic, financial, and/or political reasons.

   c) Usually the SC will be composed of established senior and midcareer faculty, with breadth across the AHC and with members familiar with and/or knowledgeable about the disciplines encompassed by the Department for which the new Chair is sought. Some AHCs have policies that specify that no faculty from the Department should sit on the SC. The reasons given for this include: 1) the importance of avoiding bias toward or against an internal candidate; 2) the need for maximum possible objectivity in assessing the strengths and weaknesses of the Department; 3) the importance of absolute confidentiality of SC discussions; and 4) and the strongest member of the Department and logical person for the SC is usually the internal candidate. Many AHCs also specify that no more than one individual from any one Department can be on the SC.

d) The Dean will charge the SC on several items, including but not limited to:

i) Possibly instructing the SC to invite external academic consultants from other AHCs to assess the Department, its needs, and opportunities—or the Dean may decide to do this this him/herself and share results with the SC

ii) Whom within the AHC the SC is to interview for strength-weakness-opportunity-threats (SWOT) analysis on the Department seeking the new Chair

iii) The role of a Departmental self-assessment, and if to be done, the contents and the timeline

iv) The Dean's plan on whether or not to facilitate the process by the use of a national search firm (NSF) to identify candidates and assist with the interview processes

v) A suggestion on how many internal and or external candidates are to be identified and interviewed.

vi) Suggestions on how to publicize the search—local, national, phone calls, advertisements, word of mouth, paper media, and electronic media. These policies and decisions will involve important diversity issues.

vii) Reviewing diversity policies regarding searches at this AHC

viii) The point in the process that the Dean and other Senior Leadership who wish to meet the candidates—first visit or second visit—and the role of Senior Leadership in interviews

ix) The point in time and in what format a candidate is to make a formal presentation to Senior Leadership

x) Informing the SC members whether they are charged to deliver the name of a single final candidate, or a panel of two, three, or more candidates

xi) The account number to which expenses are to be charged (travel, hotels, meals, etc.)

xii) The staff support that will be provided to the SC

xiii) How often and in what format the Dean wishes the SC to keep Senior Leadership apprised of the search process

e) *It is very important to note that*, in the process of giving information to candidates and answering questions, the SC should not negotiate with candidates. Negotiations occur between the candidate and Senior Leadership and/or the Dean.

f) Procedural decisions to be followed by the SC will need to be consistent with AHC policies and/or guidelines on each of the following:

i) If instructed by the Dean to utilize a national search firm (NSF), the best way to coordinate this with the SC activities and the best way to facilitate exchanges of information between the SC and the NSF

ii) Systems and strategies to identify potential candidates, especially on matters of diversity

iii) Interview formats and timing of candidate interviews

iv) Interviewing candidates one at a time on sequential visits, or multiple candidates on the same day in a round-robin type of format (usually at hotels or airports to protect confidentiality of the multiple candidates)

v) The number of candidates for the first visit and for the second visit

What should the candidate expect in the search process?

1) Prior to any candidate visits, the SC and/or the NSF will have advertised in the appropriate journals and appropriate websites, will have contacted Chairs of multiple Departments at other AHCs for suggested candidate names, and will have from these efforts obtained multiple CVs of possible Chair candidates.

2) All of these materials will have been reviewed, selective phone calls will have been made, and the NSF or the SC will have decided who should be invited to interview for the vacant Chair position.

3) A cordial discussion between the candidate and either the head of the SC or with the point person for the NSF should provide enough information about the AHC and the Department for the candidate to decide if he/she is interested in entering the process. Similarly, this preliminary discussion between the potential candidate and the SC or NSF should be a very effective first screening of each potential candidate. These initial conversations may be by phone or in person. If the decision is to proceed, the SC or NSF will ask whom the contact person should be for arranging the first visit—the candidate himself/herself, and preferred use of home or office phone number/e-mail? If the office phone number is to be used, the candidate will need to share the name and "inside number" of the trusted person who manages the candidate's calendar. The SC and/or NSF should be sensitive to and aware if the candidate wishes to remain confidential at the home AHC regarding candidacy.

4) Assuming the candidate's interest, the AHC via the SC or the NSF should provide a packet of information for the candidate prior to the first visit or first interview session. These documents should include facts on:

   a) The city or town

   b) The history of the AHC

c) The table of organization for the AHC

d) The Department's history

e) Departmental faculty and CVs of each

f) List of other Departments and the Chairs of each

g) If a clinical Department, the result and report of the last Residency Review Committee (RRC) report

h) If a basic science Department or in a clinical Department with funded research programs, the current grant funding

i) Note: the financial details of the Department and the AHC are usually not shared with candidates until the second visit

5) If a NSF is involved, that organization may conduct preliminary interviews with the candidates and/or those individuals suggesting those candidates. The NSF, as part of its vetting processes, will do these interviews to "narrow the field," as a sort of preliminary screening process prior to any candidate being invited to interview with the members of the SC. This NSF activity may speed the search process.

6) Prior to the actual first interviews with the SC members, the candidate should receive a detailed schedule for that day, including with whom he/she will interview and the position of that individual within the AHC.

7) For some searches, the first visit interviews with the SC will be conducted off the AHC campus, at hotels or an airport, with the candidate spending time with each person on the SC in a round-robin format. Usually these sessions are staggered, or held at several close locations, in order to maintain confidentiality for candidates from each other on this first visit. Other AHCs may hold the first interviews at the AHC, and these may be just with members of the SC, or may include other Chairs of related Departments. Usually these

sessions on the AHC campus will be serial sessions on different days for each candidate.

8) Very shortly after this first visit with the SC, the candidate should have feedback from either the Chair of the SC or from the point person for the NSF. In this feedback, the candidate should expect the following:

   a) Notification as to whether or not the first visit was successful for the candidate

      i) If not so, this is the end, and the candidate will be thanked for his/her interest and efforts to participate in the search process.

      ii) If the first visit was successful, the next step should be notification of a second visit. Some AHCs will wait until all first visits have occurred before starting the second visits; other AHCs will start the second visits while some of the first visits are still in process.

   b) Notification of whom the candidate will see on the second visit

   c) Inquiry asking the candidate whom else he/she would like to interview at the AHC on this second visit

   d) A detailed financial summary of the Department will soon be sent

   e) Agreement that candidate confidentiality will now be almost impossible to maintain

   f) Obtain from the candidate a list of names that the SC and/or the NSF can use for references and due-diligence inquiries

9) Members of the SC will often know colleagues at the AHC of the candidate. As second visits are planned, judicious phone calls by members of the SC to these colleagues may yield valuable insights on the strengths or potential difficulties of the candidate.

10) Big-picture information about which the candidate should ask and about which to be clear before the second visit:

   a) If the spouse or partner will be included to look at the community, schools, real estate market, etc.; possible interview needs for spouse or partner for his/her career opportunities should the move occur; or interview needs regarding children's education

   b) If the candidate will be expected to make a presentation, such as: 1) a Departmental grand rounds and/or research conference; or 2) a preliminary oral report to the Senior Leadership and/or the SC on his/her initial Departmental strength-weakness-opportunity-threat (SWOT) assessment

   c) The format and nature of the meetings with the current Department

   d) The format and nature of meetings with Chairs of interfacing Departments

   e) Opportunities for discussion of Departmental finances, and with whom

   f) If the Dean might initiate an early: 1) "let's define the sandbox of what we need and what you might want" discussion; or 2) an actual negotiating session about the Chair position (see chapter 11)

   g) Note: unlike the first visit, which is usually one day, or perhaps one and a half days, this second visit will be very intense, two to two and a half days in duration, usually with the candidate's presentation and the Dean's discussion occurring toward the end of the visit.

11) This second visit, usually with five or six candidates, will be exceedingly important for both the AHC and the candidate. If the above items have been clearly communicated to the candidate prior to the

second visit, this second visit should be smooth and very informative for both the AHC and the candidate. A great many questions will be answered for all involved. Usually by the end of this second visit, the Dean will know if Senior Leadership wishes the candidate to return for the third visit—and the candidate will have a clear insight into his/her interest as well.

12) Many AHC Deans will anticipate two or three external candidates and one internal candidate for the final third visit.

13) The third visit, for both the candidate and the spouse/partner, should be definitive. How this third visit is structured will vary from one AHC to another. The candidate should request to meet with key individuals missed on the prior visits, or with whom he/she wishes more dialogue. In some variation, the visit will include serious discussions with Senior Leadership, often as a group, and some one-on-one. The sandbox will usually have been defined in the second visit, and detailed specifics of that sandbox will be the essence of the discussions (see chapter 11).

From ethical, societal, legal, and practical perspectives, diversity is important in the search process for new Chairs. There are important considerations for both the AHC and the candidates.

1) For the potential candidate who is an underrepresented minority (URM) or a female, there may be special complexities. If only a single such person is included, there is a danger of tokenism. If two or more are included, it is more likely that the final candidate will be a URM or a female. Some generalities merit recognition.

   a) Any serious candidate for a Chair position should have had some administrative experience within a Department and/or outside the Department at an AHC and/or in some national organization(s). The same is important for female or URM candidates: similarly they should have availed themselves of all learning opportunities for leadership during their early and midcareers, so as to be well positioned when the opportunity arises to be a strong candidate for a Chair position.

b) All AHCs have a major responsibility to identify these future leaders (see chapters 6, 7, and 8). Each AHC has the significant obligation to train future potential leaders, encouraging URM and women to avail themselves of these opportunities.

c) In the search process, the AHC should make every endeavor to identify candidates who are URM or women. This involves phone calls to Chairs of Departments in other AHCs, advertisements in all the appropriate journals and websites, etc.

d) Ideally the URM or woman will emerge as strong a candidate as any competitor or as the best candidate.

e) The SC should be certain that all URM or women candidates who have potential are included as part of the first-visit interview process. If selected to progress to the second-visit process, great. If not selected, the experience will have been extremely valuable to the candidate as preparation for future such interviews.

f) For an underqualified candidate to be selected by the AHC as the new Chair solely because he/she is determined by Senior Leadership to be an inexpensive recruit is a significant error in judgment. By an analogous shortfall in judgment, for Senior Leadership to select a candidate solely because the candidate is an URM or a woman, even though better candidates are available, can be a mistake for all concerned.

To be an excellent Chair is a formidable challenge. To be prematurely thrust into such a position very often creates a lose-lose situation. The Department flounders, the Chair fails, and the AHC may drift into a difficult legal position. But should that failed Chair happen to also be an URM or woman Chair, that individual will have been labeled as "failed" or "did a poor job."

Consequently, that URM or woman will have lost credibility for any future position as a Chair. How much better the situation would have been for that URM or woman had he/she had some additional leadership training such that when becoming a Chair, success built upon success, leading to sequential leadership positions of ever-increasing responsibility.

Should Chair candidates, as part of the interview-selection processes, meet with the current Chair?

1) If the exiting Chair were successful and is stepping aside as a result of mutual agreement with the Dean, such an interview can be very beneficial. Such an interview will usually occur on the second visit. The outgoing Chair:

   a) May have very valuable insights to share on the AHC structure and vision

   b) May have very important suggestions for the candidate on what is needed (leadership, strategies, vision, resources) to move the Department forward to the next level of success

   c) May be able to give wise counsel on the Senior Leadership and the other Chairs of the AHC

   d) May be able to provide extremely valuable information and insights about the candidate back to the SC and the Senior Leadership

2) If the prior Chair were removed for poor performance, the merit of an interview with the candidate is more problematic. The outgoing Chair could poison the well and in "bad-mouthing" the AHC, preclude any successful search process.

3) If the prior Chair is not on the scene, and an interim Chair is in place, the interview by this interim Chair with the Chair candidate can pose various situations.

a) The acting Chair is a strong internal candidate for the Chair position. In this case, the potential for conflict of interest is obvious. That said, should the external candidate become the Chair, these two individuals will need to work together.

b) The acting Chair is not an internal candidate, but is a strong colleague of the internal candidate. Here also there is a conflict of interest.

c) The acting Chair is a "wise senior faculty member" who is not an internal candidate. In this case, the interview may be very beneficial for the candidate and for the AHC, similar to the results of the candidate interviewing the exiting, very successful prior Chair.

For the mutual benefit of the AHC, all the candidates for Chair, and the Chair ultimately selected, there is a need to improve the search processes that now exist for AHCs. How to meet that need is less obvious. These needs include, but are not limited to:

1) A need for more efficiency and speed in the process is apparent. In today's rapidly changing economic climate and with all the legislative actions, to have a Department (especially a large Department) lie fallow for too many months is ill-advised. With many of today's search processes, the "time slippage" calendar may exceed a year with the following sequences:

a) Discussions by Senior Leadership to remove a Chair, or discussions where a successful Chair notifies the Dean that he/she wishes to step aside, can consume one to three months.

b) Selection of a SC, charges to the SC by the Dean, can take one month.

c) Due-diligence analysis of the Department's strengths, weakness, opportunities, threats (known as a SWOT assessment), and needs by the SC or by a search firm can involve two to three months (especially as SCs are composed of senior faculty who are very busy with heavy calendar commitments, resulting in scheduling problems for SC meetings).

d) Identifying potential candidates nationally, including diversity efforts, can take two to three months.

e) The first interviews, if sequential, can consume two to four months.

f) The second and third interviews—two months.

g) Then the new Chair has to sever connections with the prior AHC and move the family (often delaying for children until the end of the school year).

h) Thus, a total of ten to sixteen months can pass for a successful search.

2) In addition to the Department drifting during the search, another problem is the loss of very good candidates. Candidate A for AHC X, who might be X's first choice after the first interviews, is often a candidate at other AHCs as well. He/she might be in the second round of interviews at AHC Y. Even though preferring AHC X, candidate A may consummate the search with Y. ("A bird in the hand is worth two in the bush.")

3) The search process can be streamlined, but this must not be done at the price of "due diligence." These due-diligence analyses must include:

a) An accurate assessment of the current Department's SWOT (see Appendix D)

b) There needs to be internal due diligence by the AHC Senior Leadership in partnership with the Department to define the realistic vision and available resources. These must align, or else the search result may be fatally compromised. As part of this internal due diligence, the search committee leader needs to be involved in frank discussions with the Senior Leadership.

c) Preliminary screening of all candidates prior to the selection for first visit. The NSF (if such a service is involved) should be able to expedite this.

d) The use of the round-robin process for the first visit should yield as much due diligence and be much more time-efficient than sequential first visits by the candidates. This latter format may have served well in prior years when the pace of an AHC was slower, but perhaps this is no longer prudent.

e) Careful vetting of candidates for second visit and in detail for those invited for a third visit.

f) There is an essential need for open, frank, and honest due-diligence conversations between the Dean and/or other members of Senior Leadership of the searching AHC and their counterparts at the AHCs of the final two or three candidates. The reason for this is that what appear to be strong candidates often emerge because of major skills and accomplishments in the academic pursuits of research, education, and/or clinical activities. These are attributes needed for academic credibility but do not convert to leadership skills and administrative prowess (see details in the chapters of Section V). These leadership and administrative attributes are essential for Chair success. It is strongly urged that external and internal candidates who are to be seriously considered for Chair leadership positions have had some significant prior administrative positions and experiences. These can be as head of Divisions, Programs, or even Departments in their current AHC and/or leadership positions at major national organizations. The Senior Leadership of the searching AHC must press the leadership team of the candidates' AHCs for an accurate assessment of each candidate's administrative and leadership efforts, experiences, skills, and results.

. . . .

Be a Leader
Make a Difference
Enjoy!

. . . .

CHAPTER 10

External vs. Internal Candidates for Chair

> *"Knowing is not enough, we must apply.*
> *Willing is not enough, we must do."*
>
> —GOETHE

The Senior Leadership of the AHC will consider several advantages and disadvantages for internal vs. external candidates (see chapter 8).

Regardless of whether the candidates are external or internal, all candidates and the AHC must recognize that Chair positions are finite in duration. And although Chairs will be charged to move Departments forward, the Chairs are stewards of the resources of the Department and of the AHC for the duration of this administrative position.

As for relevant factors for internal candidates, these subdivide into a strong internal candidate and a weak internal candidate.

1) **The strong internal candidate** is usually the result of excellent mentoring and faculty leadership training programs that have been in place for some years, which may be departmentally based, institutionally based, or a combination of the two. The strong internal candidate will hopefully have been selected after a national search. Such a national search will enhance the stature of the internal candidate as the best qualified person to be the Chair.

   a) The positives as viewed by the AHC are:

      i) The new Chair is a known quantity: personality, abilities, strengths—and also the "warts."

ii) The various AHC leaders will have worked with him/her previously, although in a different relationship.

iii) The AHC will be well aware of the quality of the prior leadership training and observed the growth in leadership skills of this internal candidate.

b) The negatives of an internal candidate as viewed by the AHC are:

i) He/she will not have new ideas brought from experiences at another AHC.

ii) He/she will not bring in, as part of a package, outstanding faculty from another AHC who are well-known to that external Chair candidate.

iii) The selection of an internal candidate may lead to the impression nationally that the AHC cannot attract an external candidate and/or there is ill-advised inbreeding. These concerns are misimpressions if the host AHC has an excellent leadership program and the internal candidate is indeed a nationally known and a highly respected person with nationally recognized academic expertise.

c) A cautionary note for the AHC is that the internal candidate should not be viewed as "a cheap recruit to be Chair," in that "he/she really wants to be Chair and is already here, so we do not have to provide a generous resource package." This scenario will most likely result in a weaker Department, problems with faculty retention, less productivity, and Chair dissatisfaction as time progresses. The AHC and the internal candidate should approach the negotiations for the Chair package with the same enthusiasm as if the candidate were coming from another AHC—and expect the same commitment to excellence for the Department and the AHC—and with the corresponding commitment of resources.

d) The positive aspects as viewed by the new Chair who is the strong internal candidate are:

   i) He/she already knows the Senior Leadership although, now it is a vastly different relationship.

   ii) He/she already will know the other Chairs; although, they will now be interfacing as equals.

   iii) He/she will know well most or all of the faculty and staff in the Department

   iv) He/she will have a solid sense of the strengths and weaknesses of the Department and various members of the Department.

   v) Because of knowledge of the AHC, the other Chairs, and his/her Department, the strong internal candidate is well positioned to develop exciting new initiatives and also further strengthen current areas of Departmental success.

e) The negative components of the situation, which may not be appreciated by the new Chair selected as an internal candidate, are:

   i) The faculty in his/her Department, because of familiarity with the new Chair, may not appreciate the new "traction" he/she has—and may resist cooperating or accepting new visions proposed by the new Chair. This may be especially true if there were other internal candidates, who may become divisive.

   ii) The new Chair, unless having a Chair offer letter with specifics, may find the Senior Leadership less deferential than they would be for an external candidate Chair and less cooperative than they already are with other established Chairs with whom Senior Leadership has worked for some time.

2) **The weak internal candidate** may be the result of a poor national search for a Department that should merit a strong external or strong internal candidate as Chair. Rather disconcerting, the weak internal candidate's selection may be the consequence of the decision by Senior Leadership to limit resources, thus precluding a strong Chair (internal or external). This leads to a situation with few positives and many negative implications. The AHC may limit the need to commit initial resources but at the cost of a weaker Department that is less productive and generates fewer clinical and/or research revenues. The weaker Department will become progressively weaker, as any good or excellent faculty will have opportunities elsewhere, and the faculty who remain are those with no other options.

The external candidate who successfully emerges from a national search will have benefits and risks from the perspective of the AHC, and there will be opportunities and challenges for the new Chair who comes from outside.

1) The benefits to the AHC by selecting an external candidate are:

   a) He/she will hopefully bring strong leadership as the new Chair.

   b) He/she brings new visions and ideas based upon prior experiences at other AHCs.

   c) He/she may well be of a stature that broadens the national and international interconnections with other AHCs.

   d) He/she should strengthen the academic Department.

   e) He/she may be able to bring outstanding other new faculty with him/her as part of a recruitment package. However, financial realities may preclude such a package.

2) The positive factors for the new Chair from outside are (note, also possible with strong internal candidate):

a) Career opportunity to move an academic Department forward to a new level of excellence

b) Opportunity to develop new programs

c) Mentor the next generation in his/her academic discipline(s)

d) Excitement in the Department and the AHC for new initiatives

e) There may well be a honeymoon period during which needed changes and advances can be initiated.

3) The risks to the AHC in selecting the external candidate are:

a) Regardless of the amount of due diligence as part of the search process, the new Chair may come with previously unrecognized or unknown problems, such as very poor emotional intelligence and interpersonal skills, lack of administrative judgment, ethical issues, and matters of personality such as arrogance.

b) Other Chairs will not know him/her and may be cautious while assessing the new Chair, thus slowing down some institutional initiatives.

c) The new Chair may take the negotiated offer letter as a mandate and hence try to move too quickly making changes in the Department. This may have repercussions not just in the Department, but also across the AHC if the new Chair's Department has essential interfaces with other Departments (examples of this would be Medicine, Emergency Medicine, or Pathology—all of which are key to successes of multiple other Departments).

4) The dangers lurking for the new external Chair are:

a) The prior Chair, if remaining active in the Department, may cause divided allegiance for the Departmental faculty even if he/she tries not to do so. It is often prudent for the prior Chair to take a one-year sabbatical, commencing with the start date for the new Chair.

b) An unsuccessful internal candidate who has a cohort of supporters within the Department may try to undercut the new Chair.

c) Other Chairs from other Departments may, while professing a welcome, try to test and undercut the new Chair and his/her Department—made more possible for the external Chair as he/she won't know "the cast of characters" among the other Chairs.

d) The Senior Leadership may renege or delay some of the financial support and resources promised in the offer letter because of emerging, unanticipated (or, within negotiations, undisclosed) financial and resource challenges imposed by events external to the AHC. The internal candidate is more apt to be aware of those impending factors.

. . . .

Be a Leader
Make a Difference
Enjoy!

. . . .

CHAPTER 11

The Offer Letter Prenuptial Agreement Clarifies the Negotiating

> *"The palest ink is better than the best memory."*
> —CHINESE PROVERB

The offer letter should define the relationship and expectations of both the AHC and the new Chair. Ideally the offer letter should be a natural extension, confirmation, and tabulation of all the discussions and exchanges of ideas between the AHC and the Chair candidate during the search process. The purpose of this chapter is to peel away the mystique of the Chair's offer letter—to define the "speed of dark."

As reviewed in chapter 4, there are great variations from one AHC to another. The specifics of these differences will often present unique items to be discussed and/or negotiated to be included in the offer letter from the Senior Leadership of one AHC that may be irrelevant for another AHC. An example is the situation where the AHC owns all the hospitals and other facilities, and thus, the single negotiation will cover all aspects of the new Chair's role—very different from the situation where the medical school and each hospital and each facility are separate corporations with separate budgets, resulting in multi-sided negotiation.

That said, from the fifty-thousand-foot view there are some broad concepts applicable to what might be thought of as the "prenuptial agreement," otherwise known as the "offer letter."

1) **There are two key concepts for a candidate to take into these discussions with the AHC Senior Leadership** as they and the Chair candidate work through the processes of the second and third visit (see chapter 9), culminating in the offer letter:

   a) The "we concept" is very important. Ideally, the goals of the AHC and desires of the Chair candidate should be aligned. This should not become "you against them," but "we" with an aligned stakeholder perspective. Such a perspective will result in an agreed-upon clear vision for the Department's goals, and also an agreement on the necessary resources needed to achieve those agreed-upon deliverables. These Departmental deliverables should benefit both the Department and AHC, and must be realistic in number, scope, and timeline. All these issues should have been part of the "courtship dance" (see chapter 9) and thus, when codified in the offer letter, should not be contentious, but rather merely making a formal statement confirming those prior conversations. If the offer letter discussions become tense, unpleasant, and confrontational, it speaks volumes that prior communications between the final candidate and the AHC have been either deceitful or irretrievably misunderstood, and that both the Chair candidate and the AHC might consider whether not to pursue an offer, but rather to abort the relationship.

   b) The Chair candidate should approach the construction of the offer letter with the realization that the AHC Senior Leadership must first consider the needs and visions of the entire AHC, and second the needs and vision for the Department within the entire AHC. Aware of that, the Chair candidate must articulate how his/her vision for the Department and the Department faculty enhances the goals and visions of the Senior Leadership for the entire AHC. Therefore, the Chair candidate should negotiate first for what is best for the institution and Department with incentives aligned, then the faculty, and lastly for the Chair himself/herself. Ill-advised is the Chair candidate who initially and primarily focuses the discussions for the offer letter on his/her personal needs package; this is a big red flag for the Senior Leadership of the AHC.

2) **What is the best purpose for the offer letter?** Ideally, the offer letter is an accurate summary of all the discussions previously held between the AHC Senior Leadership and the candidate during the second and third on-site visits, and serves almost as a checklist to be certain that all items are covered as discussed, thus avoiding misunderstanding of the prior meetings. With the offer letter's first paragraph, it is best to start with the following type of affirmation. "The AHC Name and Dr. Name have had a series of conversations and share a mutual enthusiasm for Dr. Name to be the Chair of Department X. The intent of this letter is to summarize these conversations and the understandings between Dr. Name and the AHC Name. One important purpose is to minimize the possibility of subsequent misunderstandings; therefore, if any portion of this letter is not clear or if additional items need to be addressed and clarified, the AHC and/or Dr. Name is urged to discuss this further to ensure agreement." Thus, the offer letter should be an affirmative result of prior collaborative discussions. The offer letter should: a) not be take-it-or- leave-it; b) not be the hostile result of a hammered-out agreement. Either of these will set a tone of confrontation and subsequent failure.

3) **The "sandbox concept" is very helpful.** What is this? If two children agree to go out in the yard to play in the sandbox, by definition they are within the sandbox. They are not on the swing set, nor in the wading pool, nor running indiscriminately around the yard. That said, the sandbox need not be confining. Within the sandbox, there are many opportunities for different activities. Many visions will unfold for what is to be built and how. And the "what and how" may yield opportunities for great creativity, enhanced or limited by

the tools available, the amount of sand, and the presence or absence of water.

a) Who defines the "sandbox"? The Senior Leadership and the Chair candidate both do this. Do both want to play in the sandbox, or does the AHC want to focus on the wading pool and the candidate on the swing set? The AHC and the potential Chair should each know their respective BATNA. BATNA is a term originating in 1981 (9). It means "Best Alternative to a Negotiated Agreement." If both the AHC and the candidate agree to go to the sandbox and one of them does not go to the swing set during the courtship, the prognosis is favorable for the prenuptial agreement. The "sandbox" is the outer limits of what the AHC will put on the negotiating table. The Senior Leadership of the AHC will know the limits beyond which the AHC cannot go and will know what tools are available. If the Chair candidate focuses on the swing set and the wading pool, he/she is outside the sandbox. At this point for the AHC, it is best that this candidate not be the Chair. There is no point in discussions and negotiations; other options are better. The other options might be initiating negotiations with another candidate already in the midst of second visits, might be starting the search process all over again—or even abandoning the search and combining two Departments into one, using the Chair of the other Department to Chair the new, combined Department.

b) The Senior Leadership should take the initiative to first define the sandbox. When it comes time to work out the details of the offer letter, if either the AHC or the candidate suddenly changes proposed terms on major items (i.e., one of them suddenly leaves the sandbox and goes to the swing set), the prognosis is poor for a successful outcome. In the course of the third visit, or even toward the end of the second visit, the Senior Leadership needs to make clear for this AHC how big the sandbox is, the nature of the sand that is available within the sandbox, and the possible tools. The discussions and negotiations of the second and third visit should clarify the activity within the sandbox. Similarly, the Chair candidate will know what he/she wants to do at the playground—sandbox, swing set, or wading pool. The Chair candidate had best focus on the sandbox possibilities; to suddenly decide to go to the swing set at the time of developing the offer letter is ill-advised.

c) Note: the Chair candidate is not a passive participant. The candidate also defines a sandbox and what type of sand, how much sand, which and how many toys are to be in the sandbox, and how much time is needed to work and build in the sandbox. He/she will know what the creative possibilities are in the sandbox and what is needed if he/she is to accomplish what he/she believes the Department needs.

d) If the search process and the conversations between the Senior Leadership of the AHC and the candidate have been open and prudent during the second and third visits, BATNA surprises should be few.

4) **In the course of the second and third visits and in the discussions leading to the formulation of the offer letter, there will be key items to define** in the beginning of the serious discussions between the AHC and the candidate. The AHC needs to make clear the dimensions of what is to be discussed and to frame the areas for discussion and agreement. As no two AHCs are exactly the same, and within those differences no two Departmental current states and needs are identical, the range of items to clarify are varied. Examples might be:

a) If all clinical faculty across the AHC participate in the clinical faculty practice plan and abide by that compensation plan, that fact is a given (in the sandbox) and will be part of the final letter.

It is outside the sandbox for the Chair candidate to insist that he/ she have all clinical revenue for new faculty in separate accounts outside the practice plan and external to the AHC. However, totally within the sandbox is the ability of the Chair to move resources within the Department or to ask for institutional salary support for specific needs that benefit both the Department and the Medical Center. If the potential Chair will come only if he/ she can recruit faculty to practice outside the faculty practice plan, there is no point starting any negotiations.

b) Matters upon which to agree often include which programs within the Department most need development, how many new faculty might be required, what resources might be required, and the timeline for the recruitments and for the resources. These resources should be specified in some detail— the needed infrastructure, space, renovations, equipment, etc. Those items very much fit within the sandbox for discussion and agreement.

c) If the Department is expected to increase its research profile and productivity, the resources required from the AHC, the obligations of the Chair, and expectations of the AHC are very much in the sandbox for discussion and agreement. However, if the AHC is prepared to invest $500,000, and the candidate insists on $5 million, the sandbox is obliterated and further discussion is futile (the analogy is either that the AHC is not putting enough sand in the sandbox, or the Chair candidate has decided to run around the playground ignoring the sandbox).

d) Educational responsibilities in the Medical School curriculum require agreement on the scope of those obligations in terms of faculty numbers and the time commitment for those faculty. An understanding is necessary as to whether or not any salary support is coming from the AHC or if it is all from within the Department. Again, this is within the sandbox.

e) If the AHC has major outreach into the community, the sandbox needs to include the expected role of the Department and an understanding of the time and resource commitment by faculty.

f) If performance review of the Chair is policy of the AHC, when and by whom this is done and the relationships of these reviews to Chair reappointment needs to be clarified.

5) **The offer letter should reference the need for all Department faculty to comply with the policies of the AHC, and that the Chair is responsible to be aware of these policies.** These policies need not be detailed in the offer letter, but web linkages are helpful. Examples might include such as promotion and tenure policies and procedures for faculty, compliance with electronic medical record systems, coding and billing regulations, and procedures to follow for allegations of research misconduct.

6) Each AHC and corresponding Department situation will be different, almost unique. Therefore, generalities are speculative on the types of items that are appropriate to be within the sandbox. **Usually the following items for discussion and agreement between the AHC and the Chair candidate will be included in the offer letter** (these are in random order, as importance of each may vary with specifics of the situation at that AHC):

a) The mission(s) for the Department going forward; these should be specific for academic/educational programs, research, and/or clinical efforts

b) How these Departmental missions and programs will interface with other potential collaborative Departments, Centers, and Programs

c) How those missions interface with the visions for the AHC

d) The most important concepts upon which to agree involve: 1) what are the new Chair's responsibilities; 2) what are the resources and the authority granted to the Chair to accomplish these responsibilities; 3) what is the timeline for these deliverables; and d) to whom in the Senior Leadership is the Chair accountable for each area

e) Hard-money support may come from various sources within the AHC for academic programs, research programs, clinical programs, and community outreach; these sources and the amounts will vary from one AHC to another. The candidate Chair needs to understand if these dollars will come from the hospital(s), the faculty practice plan, and/or the Dean's Office— and have the responsible individuals for those financial resources signed off on the necessary agreements

f) Incremental space if needed for these programmatic efforts, including how the costs will be apportioned, and over what timeline

g) AHC-wide leadership committees to which the Chair will be appointed

h) Reporting relationships of the new Chair to the Dean and the various Senior Associate Deans/Vice Deans if such exist at the AHC

i) Agreements on the number (if any) of individuals coming with the Chair candidate if external, and what salary and/or space/ financial resources will be provided to those faculty, indicating the yearly level and the total number of years

j) Be the candidate internal or external, how many additional new faculty may be recruited (in addition to those in the recruitment package as trailing faculty with the external candidate), over what timeline, and will there be incremental resources for this, or will all the funding have to come from within the Department

k) Special issues such as faculty appointment for a spouse should he/she hold an academic appointment at the AHC from which they are coming; special issues regarding children with special needs

l) Tenure issues: Will the new Chair have a tenured academic appointment, and if not, will tenure be considered in the future

m) The appointment as Chair must be separate from the academic appointment. Hence, the offer letter needs to contain language separating the academic appointment (especially if with tenure) from the administrative appointment as Chair, which must not be with tenure, but is at the pleasure of the Dean and the Senior Leadership.

n) In separating the academic appointment from the administrative appointment as Chair, the letter should make clear the portion of the salary that is for the academic appointment and the incremental salary for the administrative appointment as Chair. These will be separate budget items.

> *"OK...So what's the speed of dark?"*
> —STEVEN WRIGHT

7) **The Chair candidate must be economically realistic.** Economics have changed and continue to change for AHCs. This evolving and changing economic reality will enter into the search process negotiations. The Senior Leadership of AHCs are making difficult decisions on which components of the AHC are to be supported and how and with what precious resources. AHCs can no longer provide lush recruitment packages, with the exception of a very few heavily endowed institutions and/or Departments. AHCs that promise more resources than realistic will be forced to renege on recruitment agreements. The information on such breaches of commitment spreads rapidly and will seriously compromise the ability of

that AHC to negotiate in the future—both internally and externally. These negative external financial pressures include:

a) Decreases in funding for graduate medical education

b) AHC expenses accrued secondary to compliance with external mandates coming from the federal and state governments, third-party payors, and research-funding agencies

c) The emergence of increasing legal and government regulations in the relationships of industry and the AHCs

d) The fluctuations in AHC endowments

e) Philanthropy challenges secondary to economic climates and possible tax-law changes

f) Rapidly changing health-care financing

8) **Should more than one negotiation be occurring at the same time?** This is a question for both the AHC and the candidate. At any given point, more than one AHC will be seeking a Chair; similarly, excellent Chair candidates may be simultaneously looking at more than one Chair opportunity. Both the AHC and the candidate(s) should be aware that it is possible that the AHC may be in serious discussions with more than one Chair candidate—and the Chair candidate may be considering opportunities at more than one AHC. These situations are a reality. One can make a cogent argument that honest transparency is best because of the integrity implied, provided that the tone is not "play one against the other."

. . . .

Be a Leader
Make a Difference
Enjoy!

. . . .

SECTION V

The Chair's Essential Actions and Skills for the Department's Sustained Successes in the Robust AHC

> *"On matters of style, swim with the current. On matters of principle, stand like a rock."*
> —THOMAS JEFFERSON

New Chairs are awash in knowledge—knowledge of their area of research and/or clinical endeavors, knowledge of the AHC as gleaned during the search process, and perhaps knowledge of the national scene for AHCs and in other comparable academic Departments in the United States. The new leader can be drunk with knowledge and starving for wisdom—a dangerous and oft fatal state. Knowledge without wisdom can be a curse, leading to failure for the Chair and his/her Department.

Combining knowledge and wisdom can result in a powerful force to the benefit of the AHC, the Department, the faculty, and the new Chair.

> *"Common sense in an uncommon degree is what the world calls wisdom."*
>
> —SAMUEL TAYLOR COLERIDGE

Success requires creating the winning culture adopted with enthusiasm by the members of the Department and aligning the vision and missions of the Department with those of the AHC.

It is within that framework that the author offers these thoughts in Section V, based on lessons either learned the hard way or observed in others in leadership positions.

A.   Caveats for the New Chair

CHAPTER 12

Key Steps by the AHC to Mentor the New Chair

> *"We make a living by what we get, but we make a life by what we give."*
> —WINSTON CHURCHILL

> *"The achievements of an organization are the results of the combined efforts of each individual."*
> —VINCE LOMBARDI, FORMER COACH OF THE GREEN BAY PACKERS

Hopefully the new Chair will find himself/herself immersed in an AHC environment that has a program in place to mentor new Chairs. Such a program might include the following:

1) **In-house presentations, including question-and-answer opportunities,** most likely consuming a day or two, should occur in the time window of a few weeks prior to or a few weeks after the start of the new Chair. This is intended to provide a nuts-and-bolts understanding of details of organizational and support systems available for the new Chair(s). These meetings should be held in a suitable conference room, with serial introductory sessions by the URMC leadership to the new Chair, including:

   a) The CEO—overview of AHC's missions, visions, and organizational structure of Medical Center in place to achieve those goals

   b) The Dean —overview of Dean's Office, organizational structure, and academic missions

c) Hospital(s) leadership—overviews of health-care networks and payors

d) Leadership of Faculty Practice Plan – —overview of clinical enterprise from perspective of physician practices, billing and collection system, compliance office, and expense and income allocations

e) CFO and Office of Finance—overview of budgets, status, challenges, opportunities, accounts systems

f) Director of the Office of Counsel – —overview of services offered, and associated costs if any

g) Director of human resources—overview of services and policies regarding staff

2) **Utilizing resources external to the AHC,** just prior to starting as Chair or soon thereafter, each new Chair would be provided with:

a) Leadership materials from the AAMC, especially that by Biebuyck (2)

b) This volume, *Leading Department Excellence: Achieve the Robust AHC,* with particular attention to all the chapters in Section V

c) The support and mandate to attend one of the national one- to two-week courses on leadership, such as the one offered at Harvard

3) In follow-up to number one in this list, the AHC should organize a series of subsequent regular one- to two-hour meetings for new leaders. These could be weekly, biweekly, or monthly, the frequency of which would decrease as the new Chair(s) become acclimated. The topics selected and the sequence of the presentation of those topics should be tailored to the Department(s) represented by these new leaders. These topics would include, but are not limited to, all the subjects of the chapters in Section V of this book. These are the topics thought by the author to be most important.

4) Each new Chair should be expected within the first two years to take the six-month medical management course offered by many business schools (at the University of Rochester, this is given by the Simon Business School). Most AHCs are affiliated with Universities, and hopefully at the University or in that city such a course would be readily available. These concentrated courses are designed to be taken while the students work full time, with three-to-four-hour meetings held one to two evenings a week and all day Saturday. Any tuition costs associated with this should be paid by the AHC and not from Departmental income.

Although this chapter is directed at an AHC's responsibilities in leadership development for new Chairs, it is very important to acknowledge that leadership development is important for many other faculty at the AHC, for established Chairs as well as other senior faculty and midcareer faculty (see chapters 6, 7, and 8). Very importantly, the AHC must understand that this effort for new Chairs merits the approach as outlined above, and this is different from mentoring and leadership training for currently established Chairs. Each current Chair will vary in success and challenges, with a range from those Chairs doing exceedingly well to those Chairs with significant difficulties. Furthermore, those current Chairs with difficulties often have very different problems. Although new Chairs thus will benefit from a common mentoring system, established Chairs' needs will vary. That said, it must be acknowledged that many of the mentoring efforts for established Chairs will be very beneficial to the new Chairs as well, as selectively applicable.

> *"For it is life, the very life of life.*
> *For yesterday is only a dream, and tomorrow only a vision.*
> *But today well lived*
> *Makes every yesterday a dream of happiness*
> *And every tomorrow a vision of hope."*
>
> —OMAR KHAYYAM

On an ongoing basis, for the AHC's leadership support of current and newer Chairs, the AHC may want to develop a mentoring network to foster Chairs through sharing problems and solutions. The structuring of this might be varied, depending on situation specifics.

1) One example could be established in which new surgical Chairs meet with established successful Chairs to discuss common challenges and share what has worked or not worked in problem solving, be it allocation of time, salary incentive systems, budget-control problems, expense allocation, autonomy vs. team approach, etc.

2) Another example might be new and established Clinical Chairs with basic science activity meeting with new and established Basic Science Department/Center leaders to discuss challenges in extramural funding and opportunities for collaborations for extramural funding.

3) Depending on the topic(s), these meetings should include the resources of the Office of Counsel, HR, the Office of Senior Associate Dean for Academic Affairs, the Advancement (Development) Office, etc., as deemed helpful.

Be a Leader
Make a Difference
Enjoy!

CHAPTER 13

The New Chair's Key Initial Steps and the Long-Term Implications

> *"The secret to success is constancy of purpose."*
> —BENJAMIN DISRAELI

> *"Live and act within the limit of your knowledge and keep expanding it to the limit of your life."*
> —AYN RAND

> *"I put in eighteen hours a day, but I've never worked a day in my life."*
> —MARV LEVY, FORMER COACH AND GENERAL MANAGER OF THE BUFFALO BILLS (WENT TO FOUR SUCCESSIVE SUPER BOWLS)

The major responsibility and effort for a successful "Chair launch" reside with the new Chair, even with the efforts by the AHC as detailed in Chapter 12.

To be a Chair is easy, to be a good Chair is hard, and to be an excellent Chair is a challenge well worth the effort. Days and weeks will be long and difficult, but if done well, the Chair's role will be enjoyable and uplifting—indeed, a great deal of fun. How to get there has many component parts.

Real successes will come from nurtured, mentored, and encouraged faculty within the ambient environment created by the Chair, not by the Chair's personal career alone. The Chair's efforts must be directed to the larger vision for faculty development, the organizational mission, and the Department and via those efforts for the entire AHC.

> *"Watch your thoughts; they become words. Watch your words; they become actions. Watch your actions; they become habit. Watch your habits; they become character. Watch your character; it becomes your destiny."*
>
> —LAO TZU

1) **There are two kinds of Chairs**. Intra-Departmental leadership style is central to success. There are two basic leadership styles. Simply stated, the new Chair can be a dictator focused on his/her own career and interests, or the new Chair can be a mentoring leader who focuses on the faculty careers, the Department, the AHC. The Chair must put the success of the Department and its faculty ahead of his/her own academic career. Therefore key question Why did the new Chair want to be a Chair? What should be the overall style and purpose of "Chairpersonship," regardless of AHC structure?

   a) In contemplating this key distinction of individual style within the Department and within the AHC, to be successful the new Chair best remember he/she needs to: 1) create solid good interpersonal relationships; 2) create a productive ambiance both within the Department and for the Department within the AHC. Failure to recognize the importance of this and failure to achieve this will destroy/negate all of the Chair's visions he/she wishes to achieve. Productive ambiance built on mutual respect is essential.

b) This is not "the Chair show," but rather, this is "the Department and AHC show." The new Chair is well-advised to recognize that he/she is a steward appointed to advance the Department, the faculty, and the AHC. That should be the emphasis, not the enhancement of his/her own personal career and stature.

c) In a sense, the Chair is like the conductor of a symphony orchestra. The conductor does not run around from place to place on the stage, playing each of the instruments. The conductor knows what sound he/she wants from each player's musical instrument, knows when each is to be played and in what combinations, what the combined sound must express, and how loudly or softly. Similarly, the Chair leads a team and must know and direct—delegating the task just as the conductor delegates the instruments to the players. Just as the conductor delegates, encourages excellence, gives authority, and demands performance accountability, so also must the Chair.

d) In all of the Chair's interactions, the position and chances of success are far greater if the focus of discussions and deliberations is kept on *current and future patient benefit* (be it via education, patient care, and/or research—especially translational)—which means to prevent, treat, and cure today and via research and education make the patients' tomorrows better than today. This is hardly a self-serving position. Keeping this vision of short- and long-term patient benefit as the central goal will help the Chair move forward the faculty, the Department, and the AHC. This helps to build consensus, but it is best not be "preachy."

e) The dictator Chair is surprisingly common. Unfortunately, too often the author has observed, both at his AHC and at others across the country, the new Chair acts as did Dr. Seuss's Yertle, the main character in *Yertle the Turtle* by Geisel (13). Yertle proclaims, "I am now king of the mountain and of all I can see." In this modern parable, Yertle insisted that he climb on the backs of an increasing stack of lesser turtles, thus permitting Yertle to see more and more of his empire, as he became ever-higher elevated by the efforts of those below. The exhausted lowest turtle burped and the whole pile came tumbling down, plunging Yertle into the mud far below.

f) If the new leader adopts the Yertle attitude, he/she may initially be very effective with short-term results, but long-term this strategy will markedly harm the Department and weaken the new Chair's status both locally and nationally. The "lower turtle faculty and staff" will either leave or "burp." Initially, the Chair will look to be strong, focused, purposeful, and in charge. But it will not take long before the excellent and productive faculty will realize that the Chair's style and drive are centered on the Chair and the Chair's interest, precluding any meaningful role for them and hindering their career advancement.

g) This "Yertle model" eventually results in an ineffective and lonely Chair, who may have a national profile yet also an evolving ever weaker Department with little meaningful productivity by the faculty other than by the Chair, and with no possible internal candidates in the Department to be the Chair's successor. Good faculty are very recruitable and will soon leave for better opportunities. The only faculty who will remain are those 1) with little motivation, and/or 2) with relatively little talent and potential (i.e., those faculty who are less desirable and have no alternative but to remain). Although these people are less talented and with no other career options, they will still complain and either crawl within their own little nonproductive shell, or by any means available to them, actively try to undermine this misguided new Chair.

> *"Whoever would be great among you must be your servant, and whoever wants to be first among you must be your slave."*
>
> —MATTHEW 20:26–27 (HOLY BIBLE, REVISED STANDARD VERSION, THOMAS NELSON & SONS, TORONTO NEW YORK EDINBURGH, 1952)

2) As stated, the Chair who mentors and nurtures will be much more successful in the long-term. The new Chair should build mutually productive interpersonal relationships with the philosophy of: "How can I help those in my Department to succeed, and how can I move the ball forward for the AHC because of the Departmental successes?" This aligning of goals equates to a great chance of success for the Department and the AHC. This course of action will require great effort and much time expended by the Chair—time spent on others, not oneself. To do this successfully, *the Chair will need to know each of his/her faculty.* For each, what are his/her talents, goals, strengths, weaknesses, career aspirations, family situations, and motivations? How does each view his/her career to date, and what are the short- and long-term goals of each? What does that faculty member now possess, or aspire to, as a national reputation? Does the faculty member understand the AHC mission and participate as an AHC citizen? Up to this point in time, does each faculty member view the Department and the AHC as a help or hindrance for his/her roles and goals? How can this new Chair help that faculty member? Often the most important help rendered by the Chair may not involve money and resources, but rather a listening ear and good mentoring. A strong positive motivator will: value the other person; appreciate the other person's ideas; and provide an ambiance where the other person has a sense of value, respect, and input into his/her environment.

3) The new Chair has a similar key distinction to make on personal individual style within the AHC. This is similar in philosophy to the role within the Department. In the same way that the Chair wants successes to enhance all those within the Department, the successes of the Department should also benefit the AHC and other Departments. The new Chair should make it clear to the AHC Senior Leadership that he/she and the Department are firstly citizens of the AHC, while at the same time advocates for the Department and for each of its faculty. The new Chair will move the Department and faculty forward with a vision that is commensurate with that of the AHC.

4) This can be a difficult balancing task—to guard and foster the Department and Departmental faculty development and at the same time merge with the vision of the AHC (see chapter 29). The Chair must have the simultaneous goals of maximizing Departmental productivity and being a team player with the intent to fit within the AHC goals/missions/style. That is, "a rising tide floats all boats." The Chair would be ill-advised to set out to enhance his/her Department by trying to destroy another Department; to do so would most likely damage both Departments and surely weaken the AHC.

> *"Nothing can stop the man/woman with the right mental attitude from achieving his goal; nothing on earth can help the man/woman with the wrong mental attitude."*
>
> —THOMAS JEFFERSON

5) **If the Chair wishes to be successful long-term, what are the first steps, as the "new kid on the block," to get the ball moving?** *There is only one opportunity to make a first impression.*

a) *Listening tour* (**there is a reason people have two ears and one mouth**)**:** The purpose of this is to gather facts and develop insights from what others tell you—listen (*truly* listen) to others, and within that context share background and hopes. Talk *with* people, not *to* people. The new Chair had best remember that: a) he/she is "the new kid on the block" if a Chair selected from outside; and b) he/she is also a "new kid on the block" if selected as an internal candidate because he/she now has a totally new role in the eyes of the faculty and a new role in interfacing with other Departmental leaders and the AHC Senior Leadership. On this tour of listening, the new Chair should first give the other person the opportunity to share ideas and visions. That said, the new Chair should be prepared with related important questions so that key topics will receive that person's input. Depending on conversational topics, examples of such questions when meeting with **other Chairs** might be: a) "What are your visions for your Department?; b) What are your personal goals and career objectives?; c) How do your goals and those of your Department mesh with those of the AHC?; d) What do you see as the role and potential for my Department going forward?; e) What challenges do you see, both immediate and on the horizon, that concern you and your Department, and do you have thoughts on how to deal with these? f) What are your insights on my Department, and how might we most productively interface with and collaborate with your Department?" g) "How do your Department and mine best move forward the AHC?"

b) The stops on this tour should include:

i) **Departmental faculty**—all academic ranks and Divisions; if it is a very large Department with hundreds of faculty, the tour should include all the Division heads and leaders representative of all academic ranks as suggested by the Division heads

ii) **Other Chairs** at the AHC

iii) **Senior Leadership** of the AHC

iv) **Administrators and key staff** within the Department

v) **Other individuals** suggested by any of the above four groups

> *"I walk slowly, but I never walk backward."*
> —ABRAHAM LINCOLN

Within all of the above points in this chapter, there are some common and very important considerations for Chairs and their Departments. Unfortunately to the detriment of the AHCs, these considerations are often limited or even missing completely within a malignant environment of "your worst enemy is across the hall and your best friend is down the street."

1) **The new Chair needs to appreciate and develop the subtleties of his/her own position in the organizational hierarchy of the AHC.**

   a) **Mutual respect is key** and is to be nurtured by the new Chair. This mutual respect has to be earned—between the Chair and the Departmental faculty, between the Chair and senior AHC leadership, between the Chair and the co-Chairs at the AHC. Respect is worth the sincere effort required to achieve it. Once accomplished, the respect is to be treasured; for if lost, it is almost impossible to regain.

   b) It is important for the new Chair to recall that he/she has negotiated the resource recruitment package for Department first, and for himself/herself only secondarily.

   c) The new Chair should understand that he/she is a "middleperson" and will best function effectively by building consensus and the team concept, not by heavy-handed fiats.

> *"If Michelangelo wanted to play it safe, he would have painted the floor of the Sistine Chapel."*
>
> —MARV LEVY, FORMER COACH AND THEN GENERAL MANAGER OF THE BUFFALO BILLS (WENT TO FOUR SUCCESSIVE SUPER BOWLS)

2) What is meant by the concept **"A Chair at an AHC equates to middle management"**? A Chair has vertical and horizontal interfaces. The Chair does not function in a vacuum, but within a complex system of checks and balances.

   a) The Chair is accountable to those who have authority over the Chair, such as the CEO, the Dean, the Hospital Director, the CFO —in other words, the Chair answers to, and is accountable to, Senior Leadership. As part of the negotiations, the Chair and the AHC should have agreed-upon areas of responsibility, authority, and accountability, as well as the reporting structures (see chapter 11).

   b) There is another cohort, sometimes much larger, with whom the Chair will interface as equals—the other Chairs and/or Center Directors. These relationships are very important to the growing successes of the Department. Over the past years, the skill sets and knowledge bases between clinical specialties are blurring and overlapping. Examples would include Imaging Sciences and Cardiology, Hand Surgery in Orthopaedics and in Plastic Surgery, and stroke treatments by Neurology and Imaging Sciences. In basic sciences there are many examples, such as Biochemistry and Biophysics, and Immunology and Virology. And there is similar melding between basic science and clinical care. Examples would include basic science of Immunology and Infectious Disease (in clinical Medicine). These cross-Departmental relationships need time to develop and nurture, as they are based on mutual interest and common motives rather than lines of authority. They will be more fruitful with some Chairs than others, depending on the style and motives of the other Chairs and/or Center Directors. All Departments are best served by fostering these collaborative interests and skills, for the betterment of all the involved Departments and for the advancement of the AHC's missions and visions.

c) The Chair is also responsible for all those within his/her Department, over whom the Chair has authority. This responsibility includes mentoring of collaborative attitudes, not only within his/her Department, but reaching out to other faculty in other Departments who share similar and overlapping clinical and/or research interests (see "2b" in this list).

> *"Success is a little like wrestling a gorilla. You don't quit when you're tired. You quit when the gorilla is tired."*
>
> —ROBERT STRAUSS

d) The key nugget, over which the Chair has control, is development of the Departmental team. This team concept will have a major impact on the success or failure of the Departmental faculty, which in turn will determine the Chair's success or failure. Much of the rest of Section V is dedicated to how the Chair can best nurture and mentor that Department team to create the successful Department. As will be explained later in this section, in addition to all the faculty, this team will include key senior administrators within the Department—and at times as appropriate the Office of Counsel, human resources, accounting, etc. In this Department team, clearly defined areas of authority, responsibility, and accountability are very important (just as the Chair has previously done for himself/herself with the Senior

Leadership of the AHC). At the hub of the Department team will be the Departmental executive team, carefully selected, vigorously nurtured, and wisely utilized (see chapter 18).

. . . .

Be a Leader
Make a Difference
Enjoy!

. . . .

CHAPTER 14

· ·

Developing the Vision, the Plan, the Priorities, and the Strategies to Achieve Departmental Goals

"Set your course by the stars, not by the lights of every passing ship."

—OMAR N. BRADLEY

"If one does not know to which port one is sailing, no wind is favorable."

—LUCIUS ANNAEUS SENECA

Based upon the negotiations for the Chair position, the offer letter, the administrative appointment letter, what was learned on the listening tour, what insights were gained as a mentee to Senior Leadership, and all the facts the Chair has assimilated, the Chair needs to formulate a six-month plan, a one-year plan, and tentative three- and five-year plans.

"A problem well stated is a problem half-solved."

—CHARLES F. HETTERING

These plans cannot be cast in stone; circumstances change as a result of forces external to the Department and/or the AHC. Accurate facts are key; note that with time the facts of the matter can evolve and change. The author has found it helpful to consider these as rolling plans, with the longer the range, the fuzzier the vision.

The faculty need to be part of a process, evolving and nurtured toward the Chair's goals, especially if the Chair is planning to make changes that will impact the faculty. If the new Chair "struts and flaunts" the plan as a dictator, making sudden changes by fiat, he/she will only lose faculty cooperation.

A very important fact to remember is that *wishes are not goals*. To take an analogy from running foot races—the Chair might *wish* to run a marathon, but that wish will never get that distance run accomplished without the hard work of preparation. The Chair, like the runner, needs to research what is needed in conditioning, solicit advice from trainers, and establish sequential goals of training runs of various lengths, building up in distance. It is the process of *gathering facts, developing a plan based on what is learned, executing the training plan, and setting sequential goals that result in completion of the marathon or achieving the planned goal(s)*, not the stating of a nebulous wish.

> *"The height of stupidity is to do the same thing again and expect a different result."*
> —ALBERT EINSTEIN

1) The Chair first needs to recognize how much time is required for conversion of ideas into vision, then translate the vision into a plan with a timeline, and finally, develop strategies for the plan's implementation.

   a) To do this the new Chair should accept that the plans will take time.

b) The Chair should have in mind a timeline for goals and objectives with four plan time sets—"soon" (within 6 months), one-year, three-year, and five-year.

c) The Chair will recognize that the closer in time the more clear the vision and strategy, the later in time the fuzzier the view. The immediate may be obvious; the five-year is very indistinct.

> *"However beautiful the strategy, you should occasionally look at the results."*
> —WINSTON CHURCHILL

d) As step one unfolds, the results may change the strategies for step two.

e) Although this process involves stops and starts, planning and replanning, the Chair in his/her mind needs to keep focused and on track for the big-picture goals. As an example, the goal might be to build a research program, but suddenly NIH funding decreases nationally. Strategies may change to seek other sources for research support, such as to increase philanthropic efforts and endowment development, to explore relationships with industry, to streamline personnel and processes in the labs, and to look to intellectual property opportunities (see chapter 30)—*but the goal to build research remains unchanged.*

> *"When it is obvious the goals cannot be reached, don't adjust the goals, adjust the action steps."*
> —CONFUCIUS

2) As the Chair starts to move forward with his/her plan, it is very important to remember to define clearly all the issues, questions,

and challenges that arise. These situations and challenges need to be sorted by priority, which are:

a) **Urgent and important**—these are key items for the Chair to address, demanding prompt attention. That said, the Chair should not "shoot from the hip." The Chair should quickly gather the information needed. It is often wise to engage the other stakeholders. The Chair should develop the plan and have contingencies in mind should backup alternatives become necessary. For example, should the result of the Chair's plan of action cause a faculty member to depart or a source of revenue to drop, who will take over all the responsibilities of that faculty member, or what are other sources of revenue? The Chair must have those thoughts ready with enough detail to be realistic. The Chair should consult with the Dean, especially if early in the Chair's tenure and the urgent-important item/situation has impact in the AHC outside the Department and/or has financial implications.

b) **Not important, not urgent:** the Chair should not forget these, but these items can go on the back-burner list

c) **Important but not urgent:** no rush, but these must be addressed with a plan based on good information and careful implementation

d) **Urgent but not important:** the Chair should tend to ASAP, but not a big deal

"Efforts and courage are not enough without purpose and direction."
—JOHN F. KENNEDY

It is necessary for the Chair's plans and actions to be consistent with the negotiated package. It is often very prudent for the new Chair to meet with the Dean and discuss issues, timing, and general strategies. The Dean will have valuable insights and suggestions. Particularly important, this will also prevent the Dean from being surprised.

3) The new Chair should think in terms of time frames, and for the immediate and one year absolutely use the previously stated categories in "2" in the urgent-important matrix.

   a) Immediate

   b) One year

   c) Two year

   d) Five year will of necessity "be fuzzy." A helpful concept for the Chair may be the "rolling year vision" so as to be flexible as situations change. Yet the Chair should not lose sight of the big-picture longer-term essential goals.

> *"Action expresses priorities."*
> —Mohandas K. Gandhi

4) As the Chair methodically (and yet creatively) moves ahead with plans and actions, he/she needs to be sure to consider:

   a) The essential requirement is to first build Departmental consensus. This will involve the Executive Committee, Departmental culture, faculty issues, special skill sets, effective meetings, etc. (see chapters 13, 14, 15, 17, 18, 19, and 20).

> *"The best time to plant a tree was twenty years ago.*
> *The second best time is now."*
> —CHINESE PROVERB

b) Downstream secondary impacts are essential to consider. For every implementation or change occurring in the Department, there will be secondary events. These may impact faculty morale, revenues, salaries, resource allocation, changes in faculty career opportunities, etc. There may be secondary impacts with other Departments. As much as possible, anticipate all of these, and have an action plan in mind for these downstream events. These fallback plans are very important if decisions and/or actions have unexpected results.

5) The Chair's goals need to be beneficial for the AHC, the Department, the Departmental faculty, and lastly for himself/herself and family. Ideally these goals will all be aligned, as built-in conflict can be very difficult to manage. One key is to look for common ground, to align incentives and benefits. Seek allies.

Be a Leader
Make a Difference
Enjoy!

CHAPTER 15

The Chair's Personal Style Has a Major Impact on the Department's Success

> *"Strive not to be a success, but rather to be of value."*
> —ALBERT EINSTEIN

With the Senior Leadership, with the Chair's peers, and within his/her academic Department, the Chair's credibility and the opinion of others toward the Chair are fostered by his/her awareness of the big picture. It is key that the Chair be well-motivated and support what is best for the AHC as well as his/her Department. Note the great importance for the Chair to understand that respect and popularity are different (see chapter 21).

The Department Executive Leadership Team and the Department Administrative Support Team (see chapter 18) have three essential roles: 1) to serve as a creative think tank of ideas; 2) to provide a mechanism to improve the Chair's efficiency and effectiveness in leading and disseminating information to all in the Department; and 3) to serve as a confidential sounding board for the Chair's ideas and visions, by providing a valuable source of information on the "pulse" of the Department.

1) How then is it possible to **be well-respected when making these tough decisions** that are often not the most popular? The Chair's style is the key. Key style characteristics include but are not limited to:

   a) Fairness

   b) Integrity

c) Humility

d) Attentive listener

e) Ability to tell the truth calmly without pontificating

f) Being evenhanded and objective

g) Being factual and objective

h) Preventing inaccurate perception or false rumors from becoming reality

i) Giving credit to others when deserved

j) Praising in public

k) Giving criticism in private

l) Having flexibility. Flexibility is often necessary for prudent compromise, but this is *not* the same as indecision and is *not* "inconsistency."

m) Keeping a sense of humor. Clean humor can often defuse a tense meeting, especially if the humor has a point. Abraham Lincoln was a master of this art. When using clean humor, avoid inappropriate or cynical humor, which can be hurtful and harmful.

2) There is a practical and legal essential caveat about when not to meet alone: do not meet one-on-one when confronting an individual about a contentious and/or legal issue.

> *"It is wise to direct your anger toward problems—*
> *not people;*
> *to focus your energies on answers—not excuses."*
> —WILLIAM ARTHUR WARD

3) The Chair needs to **consider all the options, avoid paralysis by analysis, and make decisions**. Once the decision is made, it is essential for the Chair to utilize communication skills with the ability to explain the decision clearly without emotion and based upon available facts.

   a) Be prepared to take criticism; it is part of the job.

   b) Do not take criticism personally or get defensive.

   c) Foster discussion on the focused issue(s).

   d) Listen to legitimate concerns/suggestions. Acknowledge the value of others' opinions, acknowledge that those facts have been considered, and explain again why the decision was necessary and appropriate.

4) **Learn to distinguish/sort out faculty motives**. As an example of one way to do this, the following anecdote is relevant. This takes place at a military installation, where health providers are assessing combat fitness of young troops. A young troop is shown an eye chart, and asked which way the *E* points. He consistently gives the wrong answer. The examiner says, "You pass." The candidate says, "How could I when I can't see?" The examiner replies, "This was the hearing test." The point is, in relating with faculty or others, the Chair should observe not only the obvious, but also posturing, which can be very revealing as to true motives. This may be as simple as body language or absence of eye contact.

> *"Character may almost be called the most effective means of persuasion."*
>
> —ARISTOTLE

5) When confronted, insulted, and challenged **as a Chair navigates through difficult situations,** he/she should be objective, remaining calm and factual, *not* showing anger, even when provoked and when

to some observers anger would seem justified. The more tense and "hot" the meeting, the cooler and more objective the leader needs to be (see chapters 19, 21, 23, and 24 for many details):

a) Stick to the facts

b) Avoid expressing opinions if possible; opinions can be challenged and the thrust of a leader's goal diverted into a sidebar, whereas facts are facts and keep the leader's intent on target.

c) No personal attacks

d) Remember to keep your sense of humor

    i) "Keep it clean"—no sexual content

    ii) Never use humor to ridicule or to embarrass

e) As you work through these situations, be aware of and sensitive to those really contentious lightning rods and flash points. These types of issues can evoke deep emotions from the faculty. The Chair needs to plan carefully for these (see chapter 23).

    i) Allocation of resources—lab space, hard-money support, operating room time, clinical space and time

    ii) Salary levels, incentive plans, financial data

> *"Knowing yourself is the beginning of all wisdom."*
> —ARISTOTLE

6) When confronting a problem, a bad situation, or results of an error by other people, the Chair needs to remember that to assign blame and cast shame in public does not correct a problem that has already occurred. If the problem is secondary to errors by faculty or staff in the Department, remember to critically advise or admonish in private only. The Chair's better courses of action include:

a) As might be appropriate to the situation, the Chair can express regret, accept personal responsibility if accurately his/hers, and then move forward

b) Marshal the facts and think "solution(s)"

c) Accept the responsibility if it is the Chair's "goof," but *move on* with corrective *action*

d) Think "root-cause analysis" to prevent repeat errors and poor situations

e) Align incentives

   i) Must be good listener

   ii) Find common ground on complex issues

f) Make lemonade out of lemons

7) A prudent Chair will be cautious in whom to confide one-on-one. He/she also needs to be aware of gossip in the Department and especially to be discreet on topics brought forward for discussion at Departmental meetings (see chapter 23).

a) The Department chameleon is a real phenomenon. This is the individual who will by various techniques, including ingratiation, seem to be a strong supporter of the Chair. Should the Chair succumb to this deception, he/she will be distraught when confidential thoughts on strategies and planning are injudiciously planted not only in the Department but often across the AHC.

b) The "locker room gossip" is the individual who is not a Chair confidant, but is any member of the Department who is freely talkative. These faculty do not have the discretion to remain quiet about items discussed in Departmental meetings. These individuals jabber in the OR locker room, at the scrub sink, beside the coffeepot, in the cafeteria—often dispensing erroneous or shaded comments to the detriment of the Chair and/or Department.

8) Within the above context, how is it best to respond when the Chair is given an assignment by Senior Leadership, an assignment that usually will be in an area or areas that have many aspects and viewpoints, and often involve difficult decisions with major impact and long-term consequences? There are some sequential considerations.

a) He/she needs to decide: "Can I as Chair do this?" and "Should I do this?"

b) Is this a realistic charge, or a Sisyphean task? Is this doable?

c) Is this a task for the Chair alone as an individual or by leading a task force or committee?

d) Is this a charge consistent with the Chair's understanding of the AHC vision?

e) Will the Chair being charged with this task have access to and a reporting relationship with Senior Leadership for advice, updates, resources, and support if needed?

f) If staff support is necessary, will Senior Leadership provide this?

g) Will the Chair be given the necessary responsibility, authority, accountability, resources, and support from Senior Leadership necessary for the charge and task?

h) What is the deliverable expected by Senior Leadership?

i) What is the timeline for this deliverable?

. . . .

Be a Leader
Make a Difference
Enjoy!

. . . .

CHAPTER 16

Developing, Nurturing, and Maintaining Productive Relationships with Senior Leadership

> *"If you want to go quickly, go alone. If you want to go far, go together."*
>
> —AFRICAN PROVERB

The Chair is a key member of "the middle-level leadership team." Chairs must not function as if they are captains of their own little islands, as mini-despots. The most successful Chairs have responsive, respectful interactions with Senior Leadership, very effectively collaborate with other Chairs with mutual respect, and effectively represent and interact with their faculty and staff (see also chapter 29).

Connections with Senior Leadership resulting in productive working relationships are very important. Just as the Chair's success depends to a large measure on his/her faculty, so also the CEO, Dean, Hospital CEO, and CFO depend and count upon the Chairs. The Senior Leadership and the Chairs need to be mutually collaborative and supportive to maximally benefit the AHC.

1) The Senior Leadership's support of Chairs takes many forms, some more apparent than others. Obviously Senior Leadership controls resources—space, hard-dollar support, use of endowment funds, budgets, faculty recruiting—and, yes, parking. The less obvious support includes but is not limited to:

a) Having time to meet with the Chair when he/she needs advice or wants to alert Senior Leadership about an impending situation

b) Taking the initiative to meet with the Chair to ask the Chair's opinion or to alert the Chair about an impending change at the AHC that will impact the Chair's Department

c) Making unsolicited statements supportive of the Chair or complimentary of the Chair to other medical center leaders at the same or other AHCs

d) The favorable portrayal by Senior Leadership of the Chair's Department to their counterparts in various national organizations

2) Senior Leadership needs help from supportive Chairs who share the Senior Leadership's vision for the AHC's future.

a) The Chair(s) can often provide essential up-to-date information on difficulties on the horizon (such as rumors of issues at competing institutions), making it possible for Senior Leadership to proactively take action to avoid the problem.

b) Senior Leadership does not like to be blindsided about problems within the Chair's Department that have institution-wide implications ethically, financially, legally, and/or in reputation. Although these issues initially seem confined to the Chair's Department, they can often quickly expand to the institution. This is particularly so in cases of diversity, human resources, and intra-Departmental compliance with federal regulations and policies. If the Chair is an effective leader of the Department, Senior Leadership may rely on him/her to manage the challenge in concert with HR and/or legal counsel, but will be enormously grateful to the Chair for the alert and for keeping them in the loop. This provides Senior Leadership with the very important opportunity to give cogent advice on how best to control and solve the problematic situation and thus hopefully: 1) avoid the potential disaster if a disgruntled person or persons tries to make trouble bypassing the Chair to give disinformation to Senior Leadership, or worse yet, by going to University President or directly to the press; 2) permit Senior Leadership to proactively alert public relations.

3) In relationships with Senior Leadership, the Chair is advised to follow the chain of command and not leapfrog. For difficult problems, the Chair should first go to the Dean, rather than bypassing the Dean to go directly to the CEO. Depending on the magnitude of the issue, the Chair and Dean together decide if the CEO needs to be involved, and if so, who will present the matter to the CEO. The Dean and the Chair can also decide whether to involve the hospital leader(s) and/or the Office of Counsel and overall who will be involved in the conversations.

4) When, and for what type of issues, the Dean and/or CEO want to be informed will depend on the style of the CEO and Dean. The tighter the AHC organizational structure, the more apt the Dean is to want to be kept informed. That said, depending on the Dean's style and the issues, the communication format may range from formal meetings to a brief phone call or an FYI e-mail. It is better to err on the side of overinforming the Dean, perhaps by e-mail. At least this way the Dean is informed, and if the Dean has questions he/she will initiate a phone call or a meeting. From the personal experience of reporting to several different Deans in succession, the author has learned that the following are issues on which the Dean will want information. These matters include, but are not limited to, the list below (in random order):

   a) Suspicion of compromised research integrity—falsified laboratory data; improper human research subject consent forms

b) Faculty member accused of financial improprieties—improper billings for clinical activity or inappropriate charges to research grants

c) Faculty member accused of falsified clinical documents—operative notes and/or consent forms altered after the episode in question

d) Inurement

e) Falsified CV and credentials of a faculty member

f) Sexual harassment: which may involve faculty harrassment of staff, secretarial harassment of faculty, faculty of resident, senior resident with junior resident, junior resident with senior resident—these situations are varied and often complex

g) Diversity issues, real or perceived, usually involving issues of promotion, allocation of resources, salary levels, search processes, or harassment

5) Another purpose(s) for interaction with Senior Leadership is the possible availability of senior administrative and/or staff suport resources to resolve major Department issues that might have AHC ramifications. After informing Senior Leadership and receiving advice on how to proceed and with the blessing to do so, the Chair, if prudent, might explore what institutional resources will be made available to the Chair to accomplish the mission. Examples of these resources might include the AHC Office of Counsel, external counsel, accountants, authorization for a panel of co-Chairs, public relations, and/or incremental space and money.

6) There will be times when the Chair will be asked by the Dean to present a contentious issue or deliver a very unpopular message to his/her faculty. Should the Chair do this? Or should the Chair request the Dean be present to do this at a Department meeting? However, it is best to not "bring in the big gun" prematurely by asking the Dean

to meet with the Department as the first step in problem solving (i.e., to have the Dean or CEO get directly involved with the situation). The Chair should have the necessary faculty confidence and respect to make the initial presentation.

a) To involve the Dean and/or CEO prematurely will: i) weaken the Dean's/CEO's perception of the Chair's ability to "do your job effectively without unnecessary help"; ii) lessen the Chair's position of authority within the Department as faculty think, "Gee, you couldn't figure this out and solve it?"; or iii) very dangerously may precipitate recalcitrant faculty going out to get their own "big guns" such as outside legal counsel or go to a University Trustee "friend."

b) After presenting the issues to the faculty and having the resultant discussion with the faculty at the meeting, the Chair can then proceed to work through the issues. The Chair would be wise to keep the Dean and/or CEO closely informed as to progress; this will keep the Dean from getting blindsided by disgruntled faculty who might decide to go around the Chair and directly to the Dean. The Chair should get the Dean personally involved if the situation does not improve but gets worse. At this point, at a prompt and timely Department meeting, the Chair can wisely suggest, "I hear many concerns and questions, with a need for direct information from the Dean/CEO. I will arrange for him/her to attend a special meeting for that purpose, and urge you all to adjust your calendars to suit his/hers so we might have the optimal productive discussion including a question- and- answer session with him/her."

7) There are some issues where the Chair must promptly meet with the Dean, as ramifications are institution-wide. Directly thereafter, the Dean and the Chair will almost always inform the CEO, and the Office of Counsel will be quickly involved. Examples of these very difficult scenarios include, but are certainly not limited to:

a) The Chair has a faculty member accused of criminal activity—such as being accused or even arrested for violence, threats of violence, child pornography, rape, etc.

b) The Chair has discovered one of his/her full-time faculty is also on the full-time faculty roster of another AHC.

c) The Chair believes there is a valid reason to revoke unlimited tenure for cause.

d) The Chair sees a need to terminate the limited tenure of a faculty member (midway through a limited appointment of three to five years).

> *"Good judgment comes from experience, and a lot of that comes from bad judgment."*
> —WILL ROGERS

8) It is apparent that there will be much productive interaction between the Chair(s) and Senior Leadership. Within that framework, it is important for all Chairs, except the new Chair(s), not to be the "squeaky wheel." The new Chair(s) will often need to seek the Dean's perspective and advice; at times when the Dean is busy, this advising role can be done by others in the Dean's Office, such as one of the Senior Associate Deans (Academic Affairs, Basic/Clinical Research, Clinical Affairs, as relevant). The new Chairs will need and should have more easy access to the Dean. Established Chairs should not bother the Dean with trivial issues, as they are a waste of the Dean's precious time. By not abusing access to the Dean, when the Chair really does need the Dean's time and assistance, the request "I need to meet with you" will carry more weight.

9) In like manner, the Chair should expect to be treated with respect by all those on the Senior Leadership.

10) The overarching concept is that the Chair should have close and detailed information on what is occurring in his/her Department. Some items the Chair will solve smoothly; some matters may require advice; some matters demand the Dean be in the loop and informed. Some matters must involve the Senior Leadership from the beginning. The Chair must look upon the Senior Leadership as allies and as a resource—to be prudently accessed and wisely utilized as needed, but not so as to abuse the privilege. In short, this takes wisdom—and is part of Chair responsibility.

Be a Leader
Make a Difference
Enjoy!

CHAPTER 17

The Chair's Most Valuable Asset Is Time: Manage It Wisely

> *"The only reason for time is so that everything doesn't happen at once."*
> —ALBERT EINSTEIN

If a Chair attempts to do everything that his/her Department requires, and do it personally and effectively, the time required will exceed twenty-four hours a day, seven days a week.

Most Chairs will have a national profile and national organizational commitments, academic and/or administrative. These can involve enormous obligations of time, effort, and allegiance.

Combining the institutional obligations to the AHC, to the Department, and to the faculty—and then layering on top all the opportunities for national leadership—can result in enormous time pressure. This is then compounded by the fact that most accomplished new or established Chairs have risen to these positions by a hard-driving "do everything as soon as possible" work ethic.

If the Chair adds the need for family time and some personal time, the calendar demands become absurdly ridiculous. And with this absurdity, inevitably what follows is stress and possibly failure.

Priorities must be set.

From a conceptual basis of time control as there are only twenty-four hours in a day and seven days a week, the Chair has to make two major decisions.

1) One of the important items for the new Chair to consider is to balance his/her own time devoted to leadership activities in national

organizations versus mentoring/positioning his/her faculty for national leadership. The prudent Chair will put the career of his/her faculty ahead of his/her own. The Chair can do only so much in his/her national career—an impact of one person's efforts and time. The Chair must do some of this, but put on limits. The Chair is wise to understand that several very successful faculty with high national profiles can do more than the solo Chair as they will have a major impact across multiple national academic organizations.

2) The second important consideration for the clinical Chair in priority management is how much time to devote to his/her clinical activity. Although needing some clinical activity for credibility, every half day spent in the clinic seeing patients or in surgery, "on call," or "on service" is a half day taken away from faculty mentoring, faculty recruiting, Departmental management, leadership for new and innovative Department advances, and leadership efforts across the AHC working with Senior Leadership and other Chairs. The clinical Chair needs to realize he/she was selected to be Chair, not to personally care for the maximum number of patients, but rather to lead all aspects of the Department to maximum possible successes for the AHC internally, regionally, and nationally.

> *"The clock of life is wound but once,*
> *And no man has the power,*
> *To tell just when the hand will stop*
> *At late or early hour.*
>
> *Now is the time you own,*
> *Live, love, and work with a will,*
> *Place no faith in tomorrow for*
> *The clock may then be still."*
> —JACOB CLAYTON LEAMAN

Once these two major time allocation decisions are made, time remains the leader's most valuable asset; time is so valuable because it is in such short supply. No amount of effort will lengthen time. A leader will have more AHC and Department obligations than time available to discharge those responsibilities. There is a constant stream of individuals requesting the leader's time and attention. The legitimacy and priority of individuals and scenarios needing attention will vary depending upon the present challenges facing the AHC, the Department, and individual faculty, and the role of those individuals in either creating or solving the problem(s). The prudent management of the leader's time is predicated on putting in place a system for time management, setting priorities. There must not be a "rationing" of the leader's time based on favoritism.

Many Chairs have national leadership opportunities, and if a clinical Chair he/she will usually have real clinical expertise. These can be enormously demanding of time, and as indicated previously need to be proactively regulated by the Chair. In deciding on national activities and on amount of clinical care to render, the Chair needs to consider:

1) Is this a stable, strong Department or a weaker Department requiring constant vigil, effort, and involvement by the Chair?

2) If a strong and stable Department, is there an accomplished and astute Executive Leadership Team (see chapter 18) in place in the Department to which significant delegation is wise and effective?

3) Is the Department's Administrative Support Team (see chapter 18) highly effective and well coordinated with the Executive Leadership Team?

4) Can the Chair, whether on site or away, make time to effectively and frequently communicate with these executive and administrative teams?

Lack of time and calendar control is a potent cause of stress for any leader, including Chairs, with major detrimental impact. Without time management, any leader will most likely burn out, and for certain, the resultant stress will cause the Chair to become progressively less efficient and less productive. Mistakes will follow, adversely impacting faculty, the Department, and potentially the AHC. Faculty recruitment and retention may suffer. Issues of safety may arise in clinical areas. RRC visits from the ACGME may go poorly. Performance at national organizations will fall below expectations, to the detriment of the Chair's personal reputation.

As a result the leader will jeopardize goals, be those goals in research, clinical care, education, and/or community outreach—and be those the goals of the institution, of the Department, of the leader, and/or of the national organizations.

Furthermore, failure to address this need for time management and balance can lead to the Chair's denial of personal vulnerability and result in unconscious self-destructive behavior. Unfortunately, there are tragedies from reckless behavior, risk-taking, and poor preventative-health measures.

> *"Don't let yesterday take up too much of today."*
> —WILL ROGERS

In addition to balancing personal national activity with that of the faculty, and if a clinical Chair to control clinical efforts, the author has found eight strategies of great help in time management: 1) control the calendar, and have a trusted, experienced staff person, properly instructed by the Chair, manage the calendar; 2) *not emotionally but objectively* assess the important AHC and Departmental commitments with those of national organizations; 3) control time consumed by Chair's academic expertise, especially if clinical; 4) as detailed in chapter 14, set priorities based upon the urgent and important, urgent but not important, important but not urgent, and not urgent not important matrix; 5) have excellent executive and administrative teams as explained in chapter 18; 6) know how to delegate, yet maintain control (see chapter 23 for examples); 7) respect the concept of "personal margin"; and 8) protect family and personal time.

1) Leaders must control their calendar and daily schedules. This is not easy. The author has learned from personal experience several important facts on calendar control.

   a) Should the leader decide to *personally directly* control his/her calendar, he/she must recognize the risks involved.

      i) Taking time to manage the calendar is inefficient and depletes time available for meetings and projects, especially when meetings need to be canceled, postponed, or rearranged or when attendees need to be added or deleted.

      ii) The leader will not have time (or patience) to be gracious with disappointed individuals, listening to repetitious complaints about calendar issues.

      iii) By putting one person ahead of another on the calendar, jealousies and/or anger may be created if the Chair personally runs her/her calendar.

   b) Most experienced leaders, especially Chairs of large Departments and/or with broad institutional and national commitments, quickly recognize the need for and wisdom of someone else managing the calendar. The following points are essential to having this succeed.

   c) The Chair must meet proactively with this individual and clearly explain how he/she wants the calendar managed *with guidance* and *training* by the Chair. The leader sets the rules; the staff implements them with diplomacy—the Chair controls principled guidelines of the calendar, and the staff person manages the calendar.

d) This staff person must be aware of and understand the national, institutional, and Departmental structures, situations, and issues.

e) It is essential to distinguish among events' priorities—important and urgent, important but not urgent, urgent but not important, and not important and not urgent (see chapter 14).

f) This is not a position for the inexperienced staff person but is for a seasoned individual who:

   i) Knows the institution well, with its visions and challenges

   ii) Knows all of the Senior Leadership, all of the other Chairs, all of the faculty and the personalities, skills, and values of each

   iii) Knows the national organizations, personnel, and schedules

   iv) Must have great interpersonal skill sets to say no, to reschedule, and yet to leave everyone with a smile and accepting of the calendar change

   v) Can follow priorities

   vi) Will recognize unexpected new situations and challenges and notify the Chair and ask for guidance on the calendar priorities

g) If at all possible, leave gaps/holes in the calendar to accommodate the urgent, unexpected event, phone call, meeting, and/or crisis.

2) As indicated previously in this chapter, the Chair must humbly and wisely set his/her personal balance between the AHC and the Departmental responsibilities vs. those of national organizations (see chapters 13 and 29). This must be done objectively, without emotion or ego. The prudent Chair will put the career of his/her faculty ahead of his/her own. There are two reasons for this: first, this allows the Chair to focus on the institutional and Departmental

issues; and second, this fosters faculty careers and the national reputation of each faculty member. The result:

a) Although this may slow the breadth of the national career of the Chair, it will enhance the national impact of what the Chair does.

b) Much more importantly, it will achieve a major increase in the Departmental national profile. Why this latter? The Chair can do only so much in his/her national career—an impact of one person's efforts and time. But, multiple very successful faculty with high national profiles can have a major impact across multiple national academic organizations—and with the potential for far more national Departmental recognition across several broad academic areas.

3) Similarly, for the clinical Chair to control his/her clinical activity, it enhances the Department's clinical activity.

a) With imaginative and wise leadership by the Chair, the clinical faculty will have the necessary organizational structure, support personnel, and facilities for each to be maximally productive. This generates clinical quality and clinical volume of many faculty across many clinical subspecialty areas, far exceeding what might be the result of the singularly busy Chair's own clinical efforts.

b) By facilitating the clinical successes of many faculty, the stage is set for superb mentoring of those faculty, enhancing the national reputation of the Department in multiple clinical areas, not just those of the Chair.

4) In the strategy of calendar management, it is key that the Chair and the calendar manager recognize that matters can be important but not urgent, urgent but not important, urgent and important, and not urgent nor important (see Chapter 14). It is *essential for the staff person to know the difference* as it pertains to the Chair's responsibilities (see chapter 14). The Chair needs to stay connected with the staff

person managing the calendar so that urgent-important items take top priority and other matters access the calendar in proper priority and with the appropriate time allotted for each. If situations arise that to this staff person seem unusual, he/she should ask the Chair as to the priority.

5) The Executive Leadership Team and Administrative Support Team (see chapter 18) can be so incredibly helpful in decompressing the schedule of the Chair. The Associate Chairs for Academic Affairs, for Education, for Research, and for Clinical Affairs (in clinical Departments), and the residency Program Director should be charged with the daily oversight and management of these respective areas. The Departmental Program Administrator (as head of the Administrative Support Team – see chapter 18) should manage all staffing and financial matters. That said, the Chair is responsible and in charge. It is much like a symphony orchestra; the conductor does not race from instrument to instrument to play the wind instruments, the strings, the tympani, but the conductor is in charge, coordinating and making certain that all segments of the orchestra properly contribute with quality and are on cue, working together smoothly as a team (see chapters 13, 14).

6) Knowing how to delegate and yet maintain control is essential. The Chair should delegate responsibility, and with that responsibility comes authority to make decisions and implement action. Critically important, with that responsibility and authority comes accountability to the Chair. In busy Departments, meetings of this Executive Leadership Team can occur once a week, several times a week, perhaps even daily depending on the situations and issues. Thus, the leadership for each of these areas in the Department is aware of activity in each of the other areas. The Chair can bless, augment, challenge, or change the actions, ongoing decisions, and strategies being implemented. These same strategies for delegation techniques are applicable in national organizations as well. Depending on the national organization's size and budget, the delegation may be to other

LEADING DEPARTMENT EXCELLENCE

MDs and/or PhDs, or to senior MBA/MPH/legal experts (see chapters 13, 14, 15, 20).

7) Within the work schedule there is the important concept of "personal margin" in the organization of time in an individual's life, and this is particularly important for Chair leaders. Within the work calendar, there needs to be time set aside for the Chair to think, to organize, to be creative, to craft the key documents, to make the "off-line phone calls" to start new initiatives, etc. "Creativity time" will foster the Chair's ongoing and continuing productivity because this time will lead to innovative successes. Swenson has excellent writings on this (41).

   a) Swenson's concept is to explore ways and areas in which to set limits and controls to provide time for the self; it is all about balance in life—hurry, fatigue, anxiety, lack of time vs. calm, energy, security, and time control.

   b) Swenson defines margin as the space that exists between an individual and that individual's limits.

   c) Swenson points out: The conditions of modern-day living devour what Swenson calls margin. "Margin-less is fatigue; margin is energy. Margin-less is red ink; margin is black ink. Margin-less is hurry; margin is calm. Margin-less is anxiety; margin is security. Margin-less is culture; margin is counterculture. Margin-less is the disease of the new millennium; margin is its cure." (41)

8) Personal time away from the Chair position is essential. There are two components of this—family time and personal time. With the necessity for outside interests, avocations, and hobbies, the leader must remember to provide time for self. This is essential to avoid "burnout."

   a) The leader should not feel guilty or selfish about this self-time. This time will, in the long-term, benefit others and the institution as much as, or more than, it helps the leader. The leader will most likely be happier and healthier.

b) But, equally important, the leader's family will be more solid/happy.

c) The leader's performance at work will be better and more efficient. The leader will thus get as much or more accomplished. For the Chair to deny his/her humanity and need for self can be a prime cause of stress and even lead to burnout and/or destructive behavior. A "dead leader" (either literally dead, or markedly compromised functionally) is bad for the leader, bad for the leader's family, and bad for the AHC.

> "No man is really happy or safe without a hobby."
> —Sir William Osler

This "self-time" can take many forms/styles, depending on the leader's individuality. Some prefer this to be "time alone" to reflect and "just let go" and go at one's own pace. Other people prefer group activities, doing the activity with a "team feeling." Some "time apart from work" examples, not mutually exclusive, can be mixed and matched, depending on the Chair's personal/professional situation and the family situation (age of children, health of spouse, etc.). Time for the self will foster the opportunity (necessity) for reflection and contemplation of the "big picture." There are many possibilities, including, but not limited to, any one or combination of the following:

1) Physical exercise can be scheduled thirty to sixty minutes each day, early in the morning before others are up and before going to work, or late in the day or at noon. Studies have shown that time for this activity first thing in the morning is most reliably done and maintained long-term—a run, a swim, yoga, martial arts, rowing, biking. Depending on where the person lives and the resultant weather, the activity may well vary during the year. Physical fitness has repeatedly been shown to foster better health, both physical and mental.

2) Music—especially if daily, be it piano, guitar, violin, trumpet, etc.

3) Hobbies—painting, woodworking, sculpting, reading, bird-watching

4) Volunteer activities, such as at a Church or Temple, scouting, community food banks, etc.

5) Vacation time—ideally at least four weeks a year and can be in one block, in two blocks of two weeks, or four one-week blocks—the choice will depend on individual, professional, and family situations and dynamics.

6) Family time is very important—this is *not* to be "efficient time"! Especially in interactions with children (from the very young through college-age), the leader cannot schedule and run family time as he/she might do for Departmental meetings. Children of all ages need unscheduled time and space, if what is really on their minds is going to bubble to the surface and be expressed. It is when helping with woodworking projects, or fishing, or walking through the woods on unscheduled time that the offspring (regardless of age) will volunteer, "What do you think about…I've been thinking that… I'm really worried about…Do you think we could ever do…"

7) Faith in a Greater Being can be a rock of strength in times of trouble – —and a guiding light in better times.

. . . .

Be a Leader
Make a Difference
Enjoy!

. . . .

B. Early Issues

CHAPTER 18

Two Key Groups for Departmental Success: The Executive Leadership Team and the Administrative Support Team

"It always seems impossible until it's done."
—NELSON MANDELA

"When opportunity comes it's too late to prepare."
—JOHN WOODEN

"Gentlemen, we've run out of money, it's time to start thinking."
—LORD ERNEST RUTHERFORD

"Few things help an individual more than to place responsibility upon him, and to let him know that you trust him."
—BOOKER T. WASHINGTON

As the Chair embarks on the mission to develop the successful Department that will be sustained as such, he/she would be well-advised to recognize that in all interactions, he/she can make a first impression only once and can never take back words once spoken or actions taken precipitously (see chapters 13, 14, 15, 16).

The Chair leader needs to lead the Department as a team. The team will have many component parts. There will be standing committees and ad hoc task forces, and these groups may include various combinations of faculty, staff, residents, and fellows as appropriate to the function and purpose.

In most Departments of significant size, there will be three teams Chaired by the Chair – —the Executive Leadership Team (ELT), the Administrative Support Team (AST), and the Finance Committee. For these to be meaningful teams, the structure and culture must be a two-way street. What does this mean? The Chair:

1) Works *with* the team

2) Moderates the team

3) Leads and gives input to the team to assure the smooth progress of the Department toward goals and missions

4) Uses the team to disseminate information and vision

5) Receives and listens to input from the team

The overarching goal is to develop the winning culture in the Department. In this there are some common key elements for which to strive for all members of the Department:

1) A creative energy where all individuals are motivated to diligently and willingly work together, paddling the canoe in the same direction and sharing the same vision in an atmosphere encouraging new ideas and new initiatives with measureable outcomes

2) The insight to challenge each other's ideas, but not challenge the person; to separate the idea from the person and truly have the philosophy: "That's a lousy idea, but you're a good person"

3) The recognition that a rising tide floats all boats and that each member of the Department fosters all the other members in his/her careers

4) The sincere support of the concept that each person's actions and career trajectory should enhance the entire Department, and the Department's progress should fit with the AHC's visions for success

The utilization of teams, committees, and task groups can be very helpful. Some standing committees (executive, administrative, finance) will be permanent, while most others as task forces or ad hoc groups will be time-limited and task-specific. There are many key combinations of individuals to be formed within the Department. Some will be focused on subissues. Some will be product-focused.

The three permanent groups, so essential to long-term realistic sustainable successes of the Department and the Chair, are the Executive Leadership Team (ELT), the Administrative Support Team (AST), and the Finance Committee (FC).

> *"If you don't know where you are going, you'll wind up somewhere else."*
> —YOGI BERRA

The ELT is central and has many functions. (By the Chair's choice, there are several possible labels for this kind of group, including "executive team," "administrative committee," "advisory committee," or "steering committee"; the author has selected ELT for this document, purposefully to emphasize the roles as executive, leadership, and team.) The purposes of the ELT are to help the Chair with decision making, to participate in discussions and as a sounding board, to provide information from others in the Department to the Chair, and then to assist the Chair in disseminating information and decisions.

1) The ELT should be an extremely valuable source of information input to the Chair.

a) What are the issues within the Department from each of the areas that they represent?

b) What's going on around the AHC in other Departments with which they interface and is there information that other Chairs may not have shared? Examples would include, but are certainly not limited to: clinical program development, recruiting, faculty attrition, impending cost assessments, or research initiatives.

c) What's going on nationally for that subset of the Department, including both opportunities and challenges?

d) The ELT should provide ideas on how the Department can move the ball forward.

> *"Shallow men/women believe in luck or in circumstance. Strong men/women believe in cause and effect."*
> —RALPH WALDO EMERSON

2) If properly selected, this ELT can be a confidential sounding board for the new Chair's ideas, concerns, visions, and suggested strategic plans. The Chair should listen carefully to the feedback the ELT members provide. That said, the Chair must recognize that some issues are so disruptive/explosive that he/she may be unable to confide in anyone in the Department until he/she has carefully thought through the short- and long-term issues. In these situations, before involving the ELT, the new Chair would be wise to first turn to Senior Leadership such as the Dean, Senior Associate Deans, hospital leadership, etc., as a sounding board for advice. Remember, although such contentious issues may be new to a neophyte Chair, these senior AHC leaders will have encountered similar situations and therefore may have some wisdom. Also, with such very difficult issues, the new Chair may need support and backup from these

senior leaders: meeting with them now may facilitate this subsequent assistance, and very importantly, will proactively prevent the AHC Senior Leadership from being blindsided if the fallout from the situation has repercussions across the AHC.

3) As the Chair ponders how to move the Department forward, the ELT should be an absolutely key source of vital information, insights, and new creative ideas. Essential input comes from this ELT for planning, evolution, and accomplishing of:

   a) Departmental mission and goals: their conception, development, implementation, and then assessment of effective results and possible needs for modification

   b) Faculty recruitment and retention issues

4) This ELT should be of great help to the Chair in distributing information within the Department. Each member has real credibility among the faculty from his/her respective part of the Department and should be very valuable to the new Chair in building consensus across the Department.

5) The overarching purpose of the ELT is to assist the new Chair in leading all members of the Department—faculty, staff, fellows, residents, trainees, students—to enthusiastically paddle the canoe in the same direction, creating the winning culture.

6) Who should be on this ELT and how large will it be? Those answers will depend on the size of the Department, and whether it is a clinical Department or a basic science Department. The new Chair should appoint this ELT after completing the listening tour. With the information gained on that tour, the Chair will then have a better idea of what "makes each person tick" and which established and successful faculty are most respected by the other members of the Department. This ELT is central to the creation of the winning culture.

a) This core group should represent all aspects of the Department, and be composed of individuals with whom the Chair shares mutual respect and trust.

b) The personality prerequisites for each member of the ELT are:

 i) Members must be honest, have a vision for the entire Department, not just their areas, and be absolutely trustworthy.

 ii) The Chair respects them, and they respect the new Chair, so that they can work together productively.

 iii) The members of the ELT should not be "yes people." Although expected to be team players, they must be the type of individuals who speak openly with facts and opinions.

 iv) Each member should have a skill set essential to the Departmental mission.

 v) Members must have a vision of the entire Department functioning as a team.

 vi) Each should have a vision for the appropriate supportive role of the Department within the AHC.

 vii) Each member agrees to maintain absolute confidentiality unless the Chair instructs otherwise in particular situations.

7) The positional composition of the ELT must appropriately represent each component of the Department. This is to ensure that all members of the Department have the sense that they have a representative spokesperson at these important meetings of the ELT. The details that follow will apply to a large Department, with both clinical and basic science research. Should the Department be one in basic science, obviously the new Chair will ignore the text relating to clinical activity. Should the Department be small, the composition of the ELT will be smaller, perhaps one or two from each academic

rank, and for very small Departments may be limited to an Associate Chair and a program administrator.

a) From the established senior faculty (defined as Professors and Associate Professors soon to be promoted), the Chair should appoint the Associate Chair for Academic Affairs, the Associate Chair for Research, and the Associate Chair for Clinical Activity. In clinical Departments, there should also be the appointment of the Residency Program Director. In basic science Departments with major involvement in medical- student education and with graduate education MS and PhD programs, there will be the Associate Chair for Education (analogous to the Residency Program Director). All of these individuals are on the ELT.

b) If a clinical Department is very large, in addition to the ELT, there will often be the need for a second leadership group, also lead by the Chair selecting one representative from each Division, most appropriately the head of that Division. Depending on the agenda for the ELT meeting (see chapter 23), the ELT meeting may need to include this other group with all the Divisions represented. Usually the three Associate Chairs and the Program Director, with their established academic positions, will also be in charge of their respective Divisions. Therefore, these individuals will "wear two hats" at the meeting in terms of constituency but do not get double votes.

c) The Chair, to be impartial, should no longer represent any one facet or Division of the Department, even if he/she is a recognized expert in that field. In being impartial and fostering the necessary even handed approach, the Chair should no longer advocate for his/her area of expertise. For example, assume in a clinical Department with research, clinical, and educational components, the Chair's main expertise is Neonatology. The Chair cannot be the person on the ELT to speak/advocate for that area. The Chair will either inappropriately favor Neonatology, or in trying to be impartial, the Chair may overcorrect and not provide proper levels of support. The Chair needs to be impartial and not compromise or favor any Departmental component.

d) Key administrators (from Administrative support team, who sit ex officio on the ELT) (see Administrative Support Team information that follows below for more details on what these positions entail in terms of responsibilities in the Department mission). Each will have essential information to share with the ELT. Each will be able to ensure that the supportive administrative functions align with the decisions and actions of the ELT. Each must have a voice at ELT meetings and be respected.

   i) Program Administrator, usually an MBA or MPA, whose role with all staff is analogous to that of the Chair with faculty

   ii) Departmental financial administrator, who is responsible for all clinical billings and/or research grant administration, and who will interface with internal and external auditors

   iii) "Outside" experts, not members of Department, who sit on the ELT ex officio, only as needed depending on agenda items (see chapter 23 on meeting organization). For examples, these individuals might include someone from the Office of Counsel, an external accountant, and/or someone from human resources.

Administrative Support Team (AST): The Chair's success will be dependent on honest, wise, and trained reporting administrative staff. This AST will be led by the Program Administrator; the Chair should recruit and select the Program Administrator, whose skill sets must include those of an MBA and/or MPH combined with excellent interpersonal skills. The Program Administrator and Chair must share strong mutual trust, and must work collaboratively and productively.

1) The Chair and all members of the AST must have a respectful collaborative approach, recognizing that the administrative support's

quality and expertise will greatly enhance the successes of the Department, and the lack thereof will destroy any chance of success.

2) The Program Administrator and Chair need to:

    a) Select carefully the composition of the AST

    b) Define their roles with complete and accurate job descriptions; define areas of responsibility, give appropriate authority, insist on accountability

    c) Listen to what they tell him/her

    d) Praise in public

    e) Correct one-on-one, in private

    f) Motivate by allegiance to Department and Department mission

> *"Life is simpler when you plow around the stump."*
> —AUTHOR UNKNOWN

3) Administrative positions for the AST that the Chair needs to be certain are in place:

    a) **Program Administrator:** This individual will need the skills of an MBA or an MPH, and is the business counterpart to the Chair's MD, PhD, or MD/PhD expertise. This Administrator should report directly to the Chair, and is accountable to the Chair; the Chair should be the person doing the Administrator's performance review. Just as the Chair deals with all aspects of faculty professional issues, this person's responsibilities are with all the AST functions These AST responsibilities are human resources, staffing issues/hiring/firing, accounting, budgets, etc. In small departments all these functions will be done by the Program Administrator, who in fact may be shared with another small department. In a large Department, reporting to the Program Administrator, these areas are managed by other senior staff in the Department, such as the Head of Finances and the Office Manager. The person in charge of finance may have responsibilities ranging from research budgets, billing and collections for clinical activities, and interfacing with auditing and compliance programs of the AHC; in this connection, note that many large clinical Departments will have a budget in the many tens of millions of dollars. The Office Manager will often be responsible for hiring, firing, salary levels, and human resource issues of secretarial and clinical patient appointment scheduling personnel; in a large clinical Department these support staff can number well over one hundred persons. The Program Administrator will have an interface with counterpart Program Administrators in the Medical School and the hospital(s) in the AHC. The Chair and the Program Administrator need to meet often, at least weekly, usually one-on-one to be certain that all is in order and that each understands and agrees with the plans and actions of the other. They meet as individuals with analogous roles, function with mutual respect, and have to be able to speak openly to each other. Thus, they are in sync. If the Department is too small to justify such an administrator, then the Chair might want to combine with another Department to support such a person who can provide that excellent quality of service to both Departments.

b) **Financial Administrator:** This person reports to the Chair via the Program Administrator. Both the Program Administrator and this financial person must have absolute high integrity, judgment, and discretion. These attributes are necessary to avoid instances of embezzlement that unfortunately are occasionally attempted and must be promptly detected and dealt with. Depending on the mission of the Department (research and/or clinical and education), these budgets may be clinical billings/collections/

accounts receivables and/or research grants and facility costs. AHC and University may have various accounting systems, and this person must be facile with these. This individual should be a trained accountant and comfortable with budgets, accounts, spreadsheets, etc. If there are NIH and other similar grants in the Department, this person needs to be very knowledgeable with all the funding regulations and policies of the granting agencies. If there is clinical revenue in the Department, this person also needs to be facile with all the third-party payor schedules and policies, compliance issues, and reporting mandates. (In some large Departments, these may of necessity be two separate individuals.) The Chair must recognize and appreciate that he/she is responsible for a multimillion-dollar business that is the Department; in fact, for some of the larger Departments, these budgets are in the many tens of millions of dollars.

c) **Personal Administrative Assistant to the Chair:** This person is key to the Chair's efficiency and effectiveness (see chapter 17 on time management). This individual must have seasoned office and secretarial skills. He/she manages the Chair's calendar, scheduling, phone, travel, etc. Therefore, the Chair needs to explain clearly and educate this person as to needs, likes, and dislikes. For instance, does the Chair prefer lunch meetings, or does he/she prefer a few minutes at midday to eat a sandwich and catch up on mail and e-mails? Does the Chair favor early-morning or late-afternoon/evening meetings? How much time does the Chair need protected each day for sudden, unexpected emergency meetings/needs? If the Chair is a clinician and is also seeing patients, what types of items justify the Chair being interrupted? Once the Chair has framed these generalities, one of the key functions of this administrative assistant is to set priorities, for there will be more demands on the Chair than there is time to accommodate them. This person has to understand the

AHC, the individuals internal and external to the Department, and how to prioritize whom the Chair will see and when.

d) **Residency Program Coordinator:** If Chair of a clinical Department with a residency and/or fellowships, he/she will need a program coordinator to work with the faculty member appointed as the Residency Program Director. This coordinator is necessary for many tasks, including but not limited to monitoring the mandated eighty-hour workweek for each resident, tracking compliance with all of the other work restrictions for residents, documenting resident attendance at all conferences, documenting competencies compliance, disseminating of conference schedules, collating all the information and forms for residency applicants, assisting in the screening of these applicants, managing the interview scheduling and processes, interfacing with the Residency Review Committee (RRC) of the Accreditation Council for Graduate Medical Education (ACGME) and with the AHC office for Graduate Medical Education (GME), and serving as the "mother/father figure" for the incidental personal needs of residents and fellows in the program that do not rise to the level involving the Residency Program Director.

e) The Chair of a basic science research Department, or of a clinical Department with significant research, will need a **research administrator** to provide a much-needed source of information, supervision, and documentation on matters such as compliance with NIH regulations, requirements of informed consent in research studies with human subjects, budget and reporting responsibilities, etc.

"Always drink upstream from the herd."
—AUTHORS UNKNOWN

Finance Committee:

As is commonly stated, "no money, no mission." This is true whether the revenues are from research grants, endowments, philanthropy, clinical revenues, AHC "hard money," intellectual property, or as is most often the case, a complex coordination of all these revenue sources. Departmental budgets are usually complex and interface with AHC budgets. Just as for the ELT, this finance committee is usually chaired by the Chair. Composition will usually include the Associate Chairs, the Program Administrator, the financial administrator, and often an outside accountant. Depending on unique Departmental situations, there may also be faculty selected by the Chair because of specific roles, and/or one or two elected by the Departmental faculty.

Be a Leader
Make a Difference
Enjoy!

CHAPTER 19

Recognition and Implications of Faculty Personalities and Skills as Departmental Assets

> *"Successful people are always looking for opportunities to help others. Unsuccessful people are always asking, 'What's in it for me?'"*
>
> —BRIAN TRACY

All of the faculty should have an important value to the Department, not just those on the ELT. Are all of the Department's faculty obligations being fulfilled by existing members? If a faculty member does not have an important role, is there any justification for retaining that faculty member, or can that faculty member be mentored and become successful? Are there needs to recruit new faculty? If so, the Chair will need to develop recruiting strategies (see chapters 26, 27).

Thus, it is obvious that the Chair needs to methodically assess his/her faculty. The Chair needs to develop overview thoughts on the established faculty in the Department, carefully evaluating each faculty member. This takes time; the Chair should not make snap, premature judgments, but rather evaluate faculty skills, current roles, and potential roles.

In doing this, the Chair will need to consider for each faculty member whether to retain and promote or not reappoint. These are complex issues in which the ELT should be very helpful, and decisions will be based on resources and potential net-added value contributed by each faculty member.

Faculty need to be evaluated on intangibles, as well as objective measures such as publications, grant funding, RVU of clinical activity, etc. Each faculty member will exhibit certain personal behaviors.

In leading a Department, it is helpful for the Chair to consider both senior faculty and then the more junior faculty in terms of behaviors. Although faculty behaviors will change depending on personal motives in various settings, especially stressful ones, the author has observed certain traits that seem ingrained and predictably emerge.

First, let us consider the more senior faculty, usually the Associate Professors and Professors. Over the past forty years, the author has developed and found helpful this "fifty-thousand-foot view," which includes four types of midcareer and/or senior faculty, regardless of their primary interest and skill, be it research, education, or clinical activities. Ideally, the Chair can nurture and develop a Department composed of the first two types described next, both which are very valuable and of great benefit to the Department, the mission, and the AHC.

1) **The Superstars:** These individuals have genuine skills in research, in clinical care (if a clinical Department), and in education. Note that superstar status involves more than this triple talent. Very important, these superstars are also collaborative, optimistic, enthusiastic, creative, noncomplaining team players who do not fall over their own egos and have cultivated, or have the potential to cultivate, collegial respect in important relationships across the AHC with other Departments as well as nationally. These individuals are so crucial to retain, mentor, nurture, and develop. Of interest is that most of these superstars are low maintenance; they have positive, "let's get it done/we can do it" attitudes. These individuals are creative, and yet in taking responsibilities and initiatives, they will "respect the rules of the road" and not be devious and not bypass AHC policies and guidelines. These faculty are not common, and hopefully one or ideally several may already be in the Department. Also the Chair may

identify younger faculty member(s) with that potential and be able to mentor him/her/them to become the superstar(s) in the coming years.

2) **The "Heavy Lifters" (the Truck-Loader Workhorses):** These faculty are solid and work hard, are very productive, and are usually focused primarily in one area (or perhaps two). These activities they do superbly well, whether teaching, clinical activity, or research. They may or may not be as creative as the superstar, but they have great throughput, usually with a cheerful and positive "can-do" attitude. These faculty seldom complain, but if they do, pay close attention because the concern is usually valid. Although these faculty often have good ideas about how to move the Department forward, these individuals may often need encouragement to speak up.

> *"Potential has a shelf life."*
> —MARGARET ATWOOD

3) **The Prima Donnas:** These faculty may or may not be extremely accomplished. They perceive themselves as very special; their perception of their accomplishments, importance, and value far exceeds objective reality.

4) **The Chronic Underperformers:** These faculty are a problem and are a drain on resources. These individuals may be underfunded in research, not productive clinically, and/or not good and willing educators. They are parasites on Departmental finances, resources, and/or space. Paradoxically, these faculty are often vocal, complaining at meetings—or may not show up for meetings, preferring to stir up gossip in the halls or over a cup of coffee. They will not be recruited away. You will need to encourage their departure (see chapter 28).

5) **The "Garbage Scow":** In a mentoring leadership retreat for faculty leaders at the author's AHC (which the author was privileged to attend many years ago), the superb consultant Edward Kappus described two kinds of faculty, using the metaphor of ships (20). One is the sleek-hulled craft quietly powered and carrying its cargo through the water with hardly any wake, accomplishing the delivery of the cargo goods with almost no disruption of the surface of the water. These are the superstars and the heavy lifter truck loaders. Contrast that with the large barge carrying great amounts of cargo, pushed by noisy tugs belching foul diesel smoke, creating a huge wake with major disruption of the water's surface and perhaps even damaging the shoreline ecology. This faculty member may be brilliant, and like the barge, carry a lot of productivity in research and/or patient care. In fact they may bring in more grant and/or clinical revenues than the superstar or truck loader. They may have national prominence in one or both areas. But they are constantly: a) complaining about the Department and/or AHC, often nationally as well as regionally; b) criticizing other faculty in the Department, often behind their backs; c) being disruptive at Departmental meetings; d) antagonizing Senior Leadership; and/ or e) may have HR issues such as harassment (ie, bullying in the OR, without provocation belittling and yelling at lab personnel, or degrading residents or other trainees without justification). These faculty, although brilliant clinically and/or in research, cause irreparable damage to the Department and often to the AHC. The havoc, distrust, and anger they create in their path far outweigh the value of their productivity. These faculty are resistant to any mentoring. These faculty take far too much time for the Chair to correct the damage caused. It is best these faculty leave the AHC (see hapter 28).

Next, for faculty at the Assistant Professor level and below, there are faculty types for the Chair to evaluate as he/she considers retention and promotion with the goal to build a strong cohort of those whom the

Chair envisions can be mentored to become the next decade's superstars and heavy lifter truck loaders. One analogy the author has found helpful is teaching a teenage child to drive:

1) The teenager takes instruction from a parent and/or driving instructor and quickly learns to drive well and can take out your car alone. These are the faculty who may well become the superstars or the truck loaders; they are a joy to mentor—productive, responsible, alert team players.

2) This teenager can't find the keys to the car. The Chair gives the faculty member every opportunity, but the person is disorganized or doesn't care, and nothing is accomplished. These faculty evolve into the underachieving nonproductive burdens on the Department, often complaining and usually blaming others for their shortcomings.

3) This teenager uses just the accelerator, never the brakes, and is reckless, generating angst. This faculty member may well be quite talented and goes a mile a minute, often in more than one direction. He/she may be irresponsible by acting too quickly without considering the possibility of disastrous results with poorly planned patient care, flawed research, or inappropriate educational activity. These faculty exude enthusiasm, may try to run into or over others, and usually generate heat more than light. They often evolve into the barge scow. They may lack the focus or commitment of the truck loader and lack the innate skills and abilities and insights of the superstar.

4) This teenager can't master the steering wheel, wanders back and forth on the road, misjudges distances, and has fender benders when parallel parking. These faculty try, but just don't have the tools. They bumble along, never zeroing in on a research project or clinical specialty even when given all the opportunities. They become nonproductive.

5) This teenager insists on texting or talking on the cell phone when driving. They have the ability to be an excellent driver but don't pay

attention. These faculty are often smart with energy and ideas but do not pay attention when the Chair tries to mentor or to give advice. They are focused on what they think and what they want to do. Unfortunately, although these faculty might have the potential to become superstars, they march to their own drummer and can become very troublesome, often the barge scow.

Spanning over the top of all of the above considerations, there are two not-uncommon faculty types who may be junior, midcareer, or senior faculty—the critics and the grumblers. What is the difference between the critic and the grumbler and what are the implications for the Chair and the Department? The critic can be helpful; the grumbler is divisive. How does each impact the Department? Note that one, if encouraged, can be helpful and valuable; the other has to be marginalized or dismissed.

1) **The Grumbler** is defined by motive and style.

   i) Disagreement with leadership does not necessarily make the faculty member a grumbler. The problems with the grumbler derive from the divisive and often inflammatory motive and style.

   ii) The grumbler does not know appropriate ways to express disagreement with leadership.

   iii) Grumblers stir up unhealthy conflict. They may have good intentions, but the results of grumbling are disastrous. They chew away at the foundation of confidence and the visions of the leaders (like termites in the foundation headers and floor joists).

   iv) Grumblers can level personal attacks and often do this behind the backs of others.

   v) Grumblers' vitriol generates simmering anger in others in the Department.

vi) Grumblers "work behind the scenes," anonymous to Chair, and are not honest about disagreements, but will seed messages of discontent by these indirect means. Grumblers like this style of anonymity.

vii) Grumblers have difficulty expressing their dissatisfaction in accurate specifics but will talk in innuendos, rumors, or half-truths based on those facts that suit their purpose. This lack of specifics makes it very hard for leaders to respond effectively.

viii) Grumblers talk a lot about problems, *without* offering any solutions.

2) **Critics** have contrary ideas but are positive and thoughtful in style and motive. Working with the critic can often be beneficial to the Chair and the Department. As the author is using the word *critic*, the critic has given honest thought to the problem, is concerned, and has the confidence to go to the Chair with an often well-thought-out course of action that is new and/or different. This can be very helpful to the Chair with different positive ideas for solutions to problems. These faculty will present a cogent case openly to the Chair, ideally one-on-one with the Chair. After that dialogue, the Chair can have the critic's help with Department discussion. If the critic's ideas are not viable, these individuals usually respond positively to the Chair's contrary opinion, and listen and respect the course of action selected.

3) **How to utilize the critic to foster the mission?** For a small Department, the Chair might need an open-door policy for all faculty. For a large Department with multiple Divisions, the Chair may need an open-door policy for the Division chiefs, who in turn will need an open-door policy for the faculty in his/her Division. (In large Departments, this reinforcing of the Division chiefs' roles will avoid the risk of undercutting the authority and responsibility of the

Division chiefs. If prudent the Division chief will bring forward the critic's ideas and suggestions to the Chair.) It is important to foster the environment where the critic is comfortable coming forward with his/her insights and ideas. This is based upon and requires the mutual respect between the Chair and faculty member. This mutual respect evolves from that initial listening tour and subsequent Chair behavior and style. It is key that this critic be comfortable to come forward to permit a thoughtful, calm one-on-one dialogue with the Chair, each listening to the other to arrive at the best decision that then can go forward to the ELT. This is far preferable to the critic first speaking up at a Departmental meeting, which often prematurely splits the group into two camps, and may result in a situation that takes on a life of its own.

4) **How to deal with a grumbler?**

Consider the healthy-lawn analogy and the prevention of weeds. The best way to prevent weeds is not to attack them individually. The best way to handle weeds is a thick, healthy lawn, which keeps the weeds from springing up in the first place. If the Chair has a vibrant Department with solid faculty composed of superstars and truck loaders, the grumbler withers and usually decides to leave.

That said, some grumblers when failing just become more vitriolic and obstructionist. When the big thistle or big dandelion emerges in spite of the healthy lawn, dig it up and throw it away—in other words, remove the faculty member (see chapter 28). During that removal process, do not waste resources. Decrease salary support, decrease clinic and OR time, decrease lab space, and remove the individual from committees, etc.

Each of the valued faculty members will have particular areas of interest, talent, and skill. From the faculty types described above, it is obvious that each member of the faculty will have his/her own style of approaching opportunities, challenges, and uncertainty. It is essential that the

Chair respect faculty within all disciplines, whether clinical, research, and/or education; the Chair should not let his/her own interests and skill sets give the perception of favoritism toward any component of the Department. The Chair must not permit a "pecking order" to develop with the perception of favoritism. The Chair should invest resources of money and space into productive faculty, based on that faculty member, but not favoring one area over another because of the Chair's personal interest.

As the Chair makes this very important effort to know his/her faculty and develop a productive relationship based on mutual respect, the Chair must understand "what makes himself/herself tick." **The Chair's self-insight** as to likes/dislikes, comfort zones, and the Chair's own style of interacting with others is essential, for it is these factors that may filter or even alter the information that the Chair assimilates on the other person. Being aware of these factors will make it possible for the Chair to more objectively evaluate and mentor faculty.

> *"Search others for their virtues, thyself for thy vices."*
> —BENJAMIN FRANKLIN

There are generational differences in faculty, and situations have changed significantly in the past few decades. In working with faculty, the Chair must keep in mind that the pressures of debt are more of an issue now than several decades ago, since medical students are often graduating with major debt. These debts stem from many sources. Prominent among them are:

1) Student loans, from college and/or from medical school

2) Extra debt imposed by choosing medicine as a second career, and hence more years as a student, often with older (and more expensive) children

3) Early parenthood

4) Two-career families with significant child care expenses

5) Lack of deferred gratification (i.e., early homeownership, two cars, etc.)

The Chair should not be judgmental but rather be empathetic. The Chair might choose to connect this faculty member with prudent financial planners/advisers. The Chair should not divert funds from other Departmental obligations, or he/she would open a Pandora's box with everyone wanting extra money.

One of the Chair's major responsibilities is building the Department for strength in future years. To a large measure this will be predicated on the quality of recruited, retained, and promoted young faculty; thus, the Chair is building toward that future. How does the author decide if a specific faculty member is "excellent" or has the potential to become excellent? **The recruiting test is very helpful** (see chapters 26 and 27). These are the questions the Chair asks him/herself in applying that test.

1) If this faculty member were at another AHC, and the Chair knew everything that he/she now knows about this person, would the Chair recruit this person to join the Department? If the answer is no, the Chair had best be cautious, perhaps not reappoint or promote, and certainly be frugal in resource allocation to the faculty member in question.

2) If the answer to "1" is yes, what financial, space, and supportive personnel resources should the Chair allocate to this faculty member to keep him/her happily engaged professionally and thereby retain him/her in the Department, building for the future? A helpful way to grade the degree of excellence and/or added value this individual

brings to the Department is to ask the following question: "If the Chair were to recruit this individual knowing what the Chair does about his/her strengths and weaknesses, what level of resources (space, money, etc.) would it be prudent for the Chair to invest to land this recruit?"

. . . .

Be a Leader
Make a Difference
Enjoy!

. . . .

CHAPTER 20

Academic Prowess Does Not Equate to Business and/or Legal Skills

> *"Economics is the one science that makes astrology look respectable."*
>
> —George Bernard Shaw

Within the overall stature of the entire AHC, even the accomplished new Chair should be justifiably humble. The Chair is almost always selected and recruited to be the Chair based upon expertise in research and/or clinically specific areas. But even within research or clinical arenas, the Chair's expertise is modest in the context of the overall broad-ranging areas of expertise across the entire AHC. For example, worldwide reputation in Immunology will not translate to expertise in Biomechanics. Great surgical skill in Cardiac Surgery will not give the new Chair any stature in Neurology.

Note that a Chair's academic pedigree will not necessarily lead to credibility/success with Senior Leadership, as they are equally and most often academically more accomplished. In the new role as Chair, stature with Senior Leadership will depend on leadership skills as Chair with a balanced focus on what is best for the AHC and for the Department, especially moving forward the AHC mission and vision and in financial and legal matters.

Most Chairs lack knowledge in matters of law, finance, and/or human resource policies. Any deficits in these and related areas can be major speed bumps and snakes in the grass just lurking to bring the Chair to his/her knees, often to the severe detriment of the Department and perhaps even to the AHC. Whole new areas of nonscientific, nonmedical knowledge and expertise are now required, and the Chair will need help!

The Chair needs to remember, "No money, no mission." This aphorism is relevant to successfully managing the current Departmental budgets and is essential for strategic long-range planning. Accurate assessment of current budgets and prudent business plans for the future are of great importance. It is essential for the respect from Departmental faculty and other Chairs that the new Chair be a whiz at research, clinical care, and/or education. *But* any Chair's ego that is based on research/clinical/educational expertise can really get in the way of and be counterproductive for the Chair, the Department, and the AHC if the Chair unwisely extends that ego into matters of legality, accounting, human resources, and governmental regulations.

Ethics should be the driving force and prime principle. The intent for involving these consults in law and/or business is: a) the ethically, legally, and financially sound pursuit of clinical, research, educational, and outreach objectives; b) to be certain to maximize the successes, enhance reviews, control expenses; and c) to avoid unforeseen, detrimental legal and/or financial events. The utilization of business and legal counsel is *not* to "game the system" and *not* to see what the Department can "get away with."

Expert MBA and/or MPH skill sets are necessary, usually available for utilization within the AHC and even within large Departments or with shared clusters of smaller Departments.

The prudent Chair will also seek legal counsel proactively; unwise and poorly structured offer letters, contracts, letters of termination, human resource decisions, or reappointment letters can have devastating financial consequences for the academic Department. Even if these are backstopped by the AHC, the expenses may be cost-accounted back to the Department.

Some, but not all, of the new required skills are in the following list. The Chair needs to remain in control, but yet recognize the absolute necessity for input of information and insights from others with the necessary expertise. The Chair will need to engage these experts in business, finance, law, etc. These individuals may be the MBA Department Program Administrator, the AHC in-house Office of Counsel, the AHC human resource staff, etc. These intra/extra-Departmental individuals with their expertise will be essential for legal issues, prospective budget preparations, monitoring of financial performances, and remedial proposals as necessary. Often it is most productive for the Chair to meet with these individuals one-on-one to discuss the situation(s), gather information, and plan strategies. Usually this will then be followed as prudent by including these individuals in meetings of the ELT and/or the Department, depending on the situation. The Chair is responsible, but it is folly to proceed into unfamiliar areas unless utilizing these sources of expertise.

> *"Even Albert Einstein reportedly needed help on his 1040 form."*
> —RONALD REAGAN

1) Accounting:

   a) Institutional AHC accounting systems are often quite complex, and hence the Departmental budgets are often difficult to dissect and master.

   b) For issues related to budgets and accounting, the Chair must rely on intra-Departmental expertise from the Department Program Administrator, who usually has an MBA and/or MPH. (see Chapter 18)

If discrepancies in accounts occur that cannot be resolved by the financial expertise of intra-Departmental staff and those in the AHC, the

Chair and/or the AHC may need to seek the services of an external accountant to clarify and solve the situation. This external accountant and/or business expertise can be extremely helpful in such issues—of value to the Chair, to the ELT, and to the entire Department if prudent.

    c) Examples of some key terms a Chair should understand are listed next. Note that knowledge of these terms and their uses does *not* make the Chair an economist or accountant but will greatly help the Chair to understand what the accountants and business consultants are trying to tell him/her.

        i) Cash flow

        ii) Sunk costs

        iii) Opportunity costs

        iv) Accrual vs. cash flow accounting systems

        v) Fixed expenses

        vi) Variable expenses

        vii) Margins

> *"Accept the fact that some days you're the pigeon, and some days you're the statue!"*
> —AUTHOR UNKNOWN

2) Most AHCs have in-house expertise for human resources and for legal issues. In fact, the Office of Counsel within the AHC often has attorneys with subspecialty expertise in fields such as liability, litigation, conflict of interest, intellectual property, labor law, governmental issues, and contracts.

3) The Chair should truly appreciate and utilize these resources! If the mistaken Chair thinks, *There is not enough time for me to contact*

and discuss/meet with them, the Chair is being penny wise and pound foolish. The minutes invested with these resources may well save the Chair many hours (or even days) of time later on as he/she tries to remedy the consequences of earlier imprudent actions. Please see Section VI for case studies, many of which involve one or more of these areas.

> *"Do what you do the best, and delegate/hire out the rest."*
> —AUTHOR UNKNOWN

4) Here is a list of a few of the situations the author has seen, where the need for such expertise is essential in dealing with faculty issues:

a) Faculty in the research lab requesting lab personnel to modify research data

b) Laboratory staff destroying lab data

c) Laboratory research data "stolen" by personnel in another lab

d) Falsified operative note

e) Altered operative consent form done after the operation is completed

f) Altered research protocol consent forms after human research study is under way

g) Falsified laboratory data in publications

h) Sexual harassment—faculty to faculty, faculty to staff, staff to faculty, resident to resident

i) Diversity and/or gender issues—centered on questions of family leave, promotion, and/or salary levels

j) Threatened or actual violence in the workplace

k) Patient as plaintiff

l) Faculty as plaintiff

m) Failure to comply with state and federal regulations on: clinical billings, coding, and/or collections; NIH compliance; conflict of interest; patient safety; diversity; employment policies, etc.

n) Faculty serving as consultant for the industry that funds his/her research

o) Faculty suing over salary changes

. . . .

Be a Leader
Make a Difference
Enjoy!

. . . .

CHAPTER 21

Respect, Not Popularity, Is Important for Solving Difficult Situations

> "Everything that can be counted does not necessarily count;
> everything that counts cannot necessarily be counted."
>
> —ALBERT EINSTEIN

> "The least deviation from truth will be multiplied later."
>
> —ARISTOTLE

Popularity and respect are different. Leadership is not a popularity contest. Leadership involves moving toward the goal by doing the right and proper thing at the correct time with style and integrity, motivating others to join in the action toward the vision.

The leader who treats others with respect, listens well, communicates clearly, and is steady and consistent will garner a calm respect that with time will make those with whom he/she works content and team players.

Some Departmental or Division leaders get entangled in the distinctions between popularity and leadership. There are two general such situations.

1) The first and more common scenario occurs when those who are in leadership positions make decisions based upon what will "make

the greatest number of people happy." Often this is not the correct decision and may have untoward far-reaching adverse consequences for the AHC mission, the Department's stability, and/or the Chair's future.

2) Equally flawed are Department or Division leaders who may make the correct decision, but the implementation is devoid of consideration of those individuals affected by the decision and/or lacks effective communication with others regarding the issues and factors leading to the decision. These leaders think along the lines of: "This is the correct decision; I don't care what people think. Just do it!" They act dogmatically, sometimes rudely, without any style as to how best roll out the message with the decision and the reasons as to why the decision is necessary. Even if the decision is correct and for the right reasons, this lack of style often results in so much collateral damage that the Chair creates new problems greater than the problem the original decision was made to solve.

> *"Qi hu nan xia: When one rides a tiger, it is difficult to dismount."*
> —CHINESE PROVERB

3) Some specific illustrative examples follow, where being a leader is *not* a popularity contest, and the important proper decision may be difficult to make, involving issues as varied as income and asset redistribution, poor faculty attitude, unethical practices, inadequate Departmental resources, morals, and/or inurement (see Section VI for some case studies):

a) There is a need to use some of a Department's clinical income from all the faculty efforts in order to nurture/foster/protect faculty income for those Departmental faculty involved in teaching and/or research. How is it best to do this?

b) How is it best to resolve the situation when one of the Department faculty members is socially adept with good interpersonal skills when it suits him/her and is also viewed by faculty peers as essential to the Department's financial stability because of a lucrative practice, but this faculty member refuses to teach, has a pattern of questionable indications for surgery (according to chief residents), and uses shady billing codes (according to the business office senior administrator)?

c) What is the best course of action when the Department has a deficiency in clinical examination rooms and inadequate allocated OR time, necessitating the reallocation of examination rooms and operating room resources among the faculty?

d) How is it best to resolve the situation when a heavily funded tenured NIH researcher in the Department has recently had several DUIs and now has developed a sexual relationship with a staff person in the lab of that faculty member?

e) How should the Chair solve the situation of a faculty member who serves as a consultant to a device or pharmaceutical company, and that company funds all or part of his/her research? AHC regulations may vary from one AHC to another. What are the disclosure issues?

> *"Never ignore a gut feeling, but never believe that it's enough."*
> —ROBERT HELLER

These types of situations and resultant decisions that the Chair needs to make may often involve others in the Department and/or persons in other Departments and/or Senior Leadership of the URMC. These involvements may be for:

1) Getting all the facts needed to develop strategies and solutions

2) Obtaining advice (i.e., from Office of Counsel and/or human resources and/or CEO/Dean/CFO)

Working toward solutions may involve several possible formats and settings. When the Chair has seen one of these situations, he/she has seen one. That is, no two are exactly the same. In reaching decisions and strategies to be implemented, the Chair may have various combinations of group meetings and one-on-one discussions. In all of these, the Chair should:

1) Listen carefully.

2) Ask the pertinent questions and follow-up questions.

3) Stick to the facts gathered accurately and impartially.

4) No "shoot from the hip" conclusions.

5) As prudently as possible, move promptly so the problem does not linger and fester, but at the same time do not be hasty/premature with decision and implementation strategies.

6) In seeking information, facts, and advice, the Chair personally must assemble the information and make the decision. The ELT is usually involved in this process and can be of great value in achieving the desired goal(s).

There are some key, constant features of great help to the Chair:

1) Having personal integrity

2) Being open and listening well

3) Being fair, calm, and impartial

4) Maintaining a balance of Departmental and institutional needs

5) Keeping an appropriate sense of humor

Note that flexibility and open-mindedness do not equate to indecision and appeasement. There are occasions and situations when the Chair cannot yield/negotiate/seek consensus and will need to be tough and rigid without compromise on such things as ethical issues. For the Chair to act in the best interest of AHC, Department, and faculty it is:

1) Easy if benefits align

2) Tough if there is built-in conflict, in which situation it is helpful to look for common ground/incentives/allies but never to do so if it compromises ethics and integrity (see also chapters 24, 29).

> "When you choose your friends, don't be short-changed by choosing personality over character."
> —SOMERSET MAUGHAM

The Chair should set priorities and pick fights carefully. The Chair should keep his/her powder dry and not squander political capital. It is important that leaders are not always saying no and are not always confrontational. The most common situation in which Chairs will find themselves is one with many items and challenges to either prevent, moderate, or solve. Some of these issues will have major consequences, others less so. Some will have tight timelines, others more leisurely timelines. The Chair needs to think of his/her ability to get things accomplished like a large bucket to be sure, but that said, a bucket of finite capacity. Do not squander the contents of the bucket on inconsequential matters, but rather consider it as a treasured resource to be prudently allocated.

Leaders have to be tough. **Tough does not mean ruthless. Tough does mean ethically sticking to principles, doing the right things for the correct reasons, all the while fostering the careers of others and the missions of the Department and the AHC.** However, the truth is, the Chair can't please everybody and cannot be all things to all people. In fact, the leader who endeavors to make everyone happy will often stray from the mission and lose the majority of support. There is an interesting story involving a new church pastor. This new pastor was full of enthusiasm on the inaugural Sunday service and sermon. After the service, the head of the pastoral nominating committee (analogous to the search committee) polled the congregation as to the quality of this performance. The vote was nearly unanimously favorable, eighty-six to two. During the next year, the pastor worked really hard, investing nearly all of his energy to woo those two to become supporters and in doing so, making some poor decisions not in the best interests of the entire congregation. At the end of the second year the congregation voted on whether to renew the contract with the pastor. The vote was two in favor, eighty-six against.

> *"Always do the right thing. This will satisfy some people and astonish others."*
> —BENJAMIN FRANKLIN

In proper leadership, do not woo the few discontented for the wrong reasons; to do so will jeopardize the respect needed to lead the team for the correct reasons toward the desired visionary goal.

Be a Leader
Make a Difference
Enjoy!

CHAPTER 22

Communications—Changes and Challenges

> *"Change is inevitable, except from vending machines."*
>
> —Robert Gallagher

The younger generations of faculty, just like the majority of their lay cohorts, are electronically savvy, are used to and often prefer communicating electronically rather than face-to-face, and may think more in sound bites rather than long considerations of pros and cons of important issues.

In the last decade of the twentieth century and the first decade of the twenty-first century, incredible changes occurred in the world of electronic communications with the emergence of e-mails to the almost full exclusion of surface mail, the explosion in texting (no longer limited to tweeting teenagers), social media, and skyping. For group interactions, the commonplace conference calls or telecommunications are similarly replacing the face-to-face conversation(s).

Some of this electronic communication change is positive, in leading to more efficiency. However, the decrease in direct person-to-person contact has had some deleterious effects and untoward consequences. A great deal is communicated via body language, and conversation nuance is lost in the electronic connection.

What is the prudent role for the electronic format? When should the Chair strive for meetings that are face-to-face in the same room vs. some form of electronic connection? The more the purpose of the interaction is to communicate facts without discussion or input, the greater the value of the impersonal e-mail, by which a great deal of factual information can be very efficiently distributed to a great many recipients. The usefulness of electronic communication is inversely proportional to the need for discussion, for consensus development, and for decision making on important issues. Electronic communications take away much of the opportunity to observe nonverbal clues and subtle body language.

The role of emerging communication venues/systems will have an impact in all of the new Chair's communications, be these communication interactions one-on-one or in groups. The new Chair has three directions of interpersonal interaction. In all of these venues, there are several constants of style the new Chair (and all Chairs) should demonstrate—calmness, integrity, knowledgeable of the facts, listening, speaking thoughtfully, etc. These communication relationships are:

1) Vertical with the Senior Leadership to whom he/she reports

2) Vertical with those who report to the Chair

3) Horizontal with peer Chairs

There are many settings for interactions, all of which involve communicating, but not all are suitable for the electronic formats. Meeting varieties include: one-on-one, the Chair with a small subgroup, and the Chair with a large group (i.e., all the other Chairs or all of the Division chiefs in his/her Department). The suitability of the electronic format is inversely proportional to the need for confidentiality, the need for open dialogue and discussion leading to later decisions, and the need for persuasion (see also chapters 21, 23).

The role of the Chair varies; there are meetings where the Chair is in charge and running the meeting vs. meetings where the Chair is part of a larger group when the meeting has been called by and is being run by someone else (see also chapter 23).

Electronic communications can take several forms, but all put a "visual distance" between the leader and others at the meeting.

1) Conference call: Participants can stay involved, but oftentimes those "in attendance" will turn off the speaker of their speaker phone and do desk work or even hold another simultaneous meeting. Those participants who remain engaged have to rely on voice inflections to augment the words and miss all the visual clues as to engagement and body language that convey real opinions.

2) "Social" media that is visual, such as Skype or closed-circuit TV, is probably better than the conference call, in that visual clues exist to convey real thoughts, and obviously, participants cannot turn off sound and visual to permit desk work or other simultaneous meetings. But this visual electronic format still lacks the personal sense of warmth (or indifference) among participants.

3) The website or e-mail notification information sent out as "for your information" is common, but it can carry the message, "This is decided; I do not care about your input. This is what we are going to do." Even if responses are requested, participation will be incomplete, either from a personal disconnect, or because the person who might respond in the setting of a meeting will hesitate to make e-mail or web-based response out of concern that "it might go viral" by being forwarded to others who are not included in the "electronic meeting."

4) The electronic interfaces such as Twitter, Facebook, and instant messaging are more suited for gossip, not the serious dialogue of the AHC, especially when complex issues are involved that require substantive (and often subtle) thought, not just the sound bite.

The digital network has a place and a purpose, but it has limitations. Mace emphasizes (22):

1) Why digital networking is important and what it can do:

a) Impersonal maximization of data compilation and data sharing

b) Provide constant information updates in a setting where there is a need for this

c) Ability to share information across a group or groups, where discussion and deliberation are not required

d) Control/expedite information flow

2) As AHCs are in the "people business," here is what digital networks cannot do:

a) Ask the right questions—computers are data, so key personnel can access data, but only people can ask the correct questions, and face-to-face dialogue fosters asking the in depth question

b) Bricks, computers, and iPads do not see patients, do not do research, and cannot replace face-to-face human interactions among layers of leadership, between patient and doctor, and between physician and NP/PA. Computers cannot replace the research conference where research faculty and graduate students share ideas, dialogue, look at data, and challenge each other face-to-face—and in the process spawn new ideas from the challenges while building the essential interpersonal team relationships.

The new Chair should not underestimate the great intangible value of the one-on-one and group face-to-face meetings for body language, visual clues, and eye contact, all of which enhance the development of the faculty understanding each other and developing collegiality.

1) As an example of this importance of nonverbal communications, the author clearly recalls a series of meetings involving about twenty faculty. One faculty member, who in one-on-one settings had been very supportive and espoused plan A, exhibited severe body language in the larger group indicating amazing hostility against any "A," even though his words were neutral when it looked as if the

group was moving to consensus in favor of the plan. Actions speak louder than words and often are very helpful in sorting out whom the Chair can trust and count on for support and who may be very devious and undermining.

2) Power of group pressure and group dynamics can be very important. The more complex the decision and the more convoluted the discussion to reach a decision, the greater the value of face-to-face meetings. That said, face-to-face meetings are not helpful unless proper planning of these meetings is conducted (see chapters 21, 23).

3) There is the need to avoid making communication formats a generational issue. The decision on electronic vs. face-to-face should be driven by the details of the task requiring the meeting. If one or more members of the group are not versed in the electronic world, either plan for face-to-face interactions or provide those faculty with the necessary technology education and support.

4) If the decision is to not have a virtual meeting or use a digital network but rather to have a face-to-face meeting, be it one-on-one or in a group, all participants should avoid the following actions. Participating in or using these behaviors will poison the meeting ambiance and decrease the chance of successful consensus and productive outcome (see chapters 21, 23).

   a) Looking at cell phone, answering e-mails, etc., on smartphone during the meeting

   b) Cutting sarcasm

   c) Dirty jokes

   d) Comments that are insensitive to race, to gender, and to sexual orientation

   e) Exhibiting inappropriate emotion—anger, arrogance

   f) Swearing, dirty language

g) Body language such as sitting with arms folded, avoiding eye-to-eye contact

h) All participants should sit in chairs of the same type and size; the leader should avoid the big-chair syndrome (i.e., throne complex), looking down at those he/she is "addressing."

5) Positive steps to control the meeting (see also chapter 23):

a) Stick to the facts, and avoid emotion

b) Listen carefully

c) Speak clearly, firmly, but gently

d) Be genuine and appropriately cordial

e) Appropriate occasional use of clean humor

f) Be dignified, but not aloof

g) Recognize that appropriate clothing indicates respect for the other person

6) Issues from generational differences that may impact communication situations.

a) The two-career family can impose significant time constraints, such as need to defer to the spousal schedule, to accommodate sick children, etc. In these situations, the engaged and involved faculty member who needs and wants to be involved may be able to productively participate in meetings, but at a distance by calling into the meeting via conference phone or even via electronic tools. That said, that person's integration into the discussions and conclusions may well be decreased, and even necessitate a one-on-one follow-up meeting with the Chair to avoid misunderstandings of the decisions and implementation of those decisions.

b) There are interests other than career that, depending on dynamics, may merit utilization of electronic tools. As Chair, it may take considerable wisdom in how to best keep the time-challenged faculty member involved as much as would be ideal.

These issues are more common now with two-career families and include the need for family leave for male and female for birth or adoption, problems with aging parents, and difficult health issues with spouse, children, and/or grandchildren—and at times the faculty member him/herself.

Be a Leader
Make a Difference
Enjoy!

CHAPTER 23

Productive Meetings—Make This a Reality, Not an Oxymoron

"Give me six hours to chop down a tree and I will spend the first four sharpening the axe."

—ABRAHAM LINCOLN

Wisely planned, properly run, and well-followed-up meetings are extremely valuable and important. Unplanned, uncontrolled, and not-followed-up meetings are a waste of everyone's time and are usually counterproductive.

Why have meetings and what are some important purposes?

- Orchestrate and implement the leadership ideas, plans, and strategies from the ELT (executive Leadership Team, see chapter 18) by sharing them with the Department and getting from the faculty valuable feedback and further suggestions

- Build consensus within Department/Center and avoid dissension

- For the Chair to disseminate information

- Get helpful input from faculty on important issues and decisions that the Chair is encountering

- Obtain information and insights from faculty on what is occurring elsewhere in the AHC

What will make a meeting successful?

- Clearly defined purpose(s)

- Good meeting leadership skills

- Preparation prior to the meeting

- Appropriate follow-up after the meeting

For the Chair of the Department, the time spent prior to and after the meeting will usually be greater than that consumed by the meeting itself. Prior to the larger targeted meeting (Departmental or divisional), several decisions and actions must occur.

1) Is this a regularly scheduled meeting or a special one-time meeting? If a regular meeting, what items from prior meetings are still pending decisions? If this is a special meeting, what is its purpose?

2) Scheduling of regular recurrent meetings:

   a) Regular recurrent meetings should be scheduled on the day of week and at the time of day when the maximum attendance can occur. For the proposed recurrent meetings (i.e., daily, weekly, or monthly) the new Chair should take a poll prior to the first meeting—best day, best time, etc.—and try to accommodate as many as possible without change of calendars, and then ask others to try to change individual calendars to attend. Therefore, early on there is a need to get agreement by the most possible members of the Department for the day of week and time of day if a weekly meeting, and if once a month, get agreement on such a time as "the third Thursday of every month at 7:30 a.m."

   b) For those individuals unable to attend for legitimate conflicts, work with them to see if with assistance (such as altering clinic times, etc.) they may also be able to attend. Should that not be possible, the Chair should decide—can an alternate be sent? If the person needs an alternate for all meetings, this merits a meeting to explore the "why." Does this indicate a lack of commitment or interest? If so, this may have implications beyond meeting attendance, indicating suboptimal involvement and commitment to the mission.

3) Scheduling of a special extra (i.e., one-time) meeting.

a) This should not be abused by being done frequently. Is the topic driving the need for this special meeting so urgent and so important that it cannot wait for the next regularly scheduled meeting? Almost by definition, these unscheduled meetings must be both urgent and important (see chapter 14). A need for unscheduled special meetings will not happen often if regular meetings are held weekly—and some major leadership meetings may even be held daily, so special meetings will not be common at that level.

b) When the notice is sent for this special meeting, try to have it at a time of the day when the greatest number of faculty are able to attend—as an example, at 6:30 a.m. or 6:00 p.m.

If the early time, provide coffee, juice, and bagels as a breakfast meeting for those faculty on the way to their scheduled days. If the late time, provide cheese/crackers and sodas for those faculty who may well have not had lunch due to hectic day schedules.

Should the meeting be at noon, provide lunch.

In the notice of the meeting it may or may not be wise to include the topic and reason. Not infrequently the topic and reason for urgent important meetings may be for a confidential and/or con- troversial matter(s) and/or of a potentially inflammatory nature. In those instances where explanations are necessary to defuse the tension, it is best to introduce the topic and agenda at the time of the meeting when the information can be framed by the leader's introductory comments, so the leader can be absolutely certain as to accuracy and innuendo.

4) Meeting no-no's that will with time guarantee poor attendance in the future (for both regular and special meetings):

a) Start meetings late

b) Let meetings run long and finish late

c) Have no organized agenda

d) Not have any items worth discussing and therefore wasting faculty time

e) Letting discussions wander off the focus of the topic

f) Failure for follow-up on decisions and/or actions after the meeting

5) For any meeting, the Chair must decide the purpose(s) of meeting. If there are no items meriting a meeting, cancel! Nothing will turn off faculty faster than holding meetings without purpose. Therefore, prior to the meeting, the Chair should decide proactively:

a) What are the items to go on the agenda?

b) How best to sequence the items on the agenda? Will the results from one item influence subsequent discussion on other items and if so, positively or negatively?

c) What is the priority of these items?

d) What is the outcome intended for each of these items?

e) Which members of the Department or Center will have insights/ comments that might be helpful? Be certain to not just hear their comments but to understand "the why for what is said."

f) Are there controversial items to be on agenda, and if so, who at the meeting might be opposed, and who might be supportive? If an individual is known to be strongly opposed, should the Chair meet with this individual(s) one-on-one prior to meeting when there are controversial items to be discussed? If so, the Chair needs to carefully construct the meeting with a firm outcome in mind.

g) Are there people external to the Department/division who need to be included/invited, and if so why and with what intended outcome?

6) In summary, regular meeting strategies include:

a) Meetings must have purposes that make sense and resonate with faculty in Department/Center

b) Faculty must know that their input is important and will be given due consideration

c) Sequential, regularly scheduled meetings should have a continuity from one meeting to the next (see below under organization of agendas)

d) Faculty need to understand the differences in items for information vs. items for discussion vs. items for decision.

> *"It is the business of the teacher to arouse curiosity, not to satisfy it. The measure of a teacher's success lies not in his [her] own ideas but in those which radiate from his [her] pupils."*
> —HARVEY CUSHING, CONSECRATIO MEDICI

7) As detailed above, since constructing the agenda prior to the meeting is very important, how can this best be accomplished? The author has found the best way to organize an agenda is into four parts—items for information, items for discussion, items for action, follow-up planning. Prior input from the ELT for agenda items can be very helpful.

a) **Items for information**: These are just that, items for information, not for discussion. Although tempting to send these electronically prior to the meeting, the author advises against that action. The reason is that faculty may need clarification or have questions on such as timing of implementation. Examples of items for information might be:

    i) An edict coming from Senior Leadership, such as the AHC will designate Presidents Day as an institutional holiday

    ii) A decision made at prior Department meeting has been implemented

    iii) The University Trustees have approved Dr. X's promotion to Associate Professor

    iv) The AHC has added (or will delete) a pretax item to the benefits package

b) **Items for discussion**: The discussions should be based on facts, with opinions explained with facts and not emotion. Examples of discussion items are:

    i) To obtain ideas from faculty on possible changes in residents' clinical rotations or on possible ways to improve mentoring of PhD students

    ii) Impending federal and/or state legislation, and what input would they like to see the Department provide to the AHC's Senior Leadership

    iii) To obtain faculty suggestions on how to best allocate Department expenses

    iv) Get suggested names for faculty who might serve on AHC committees

Directly after the discussions it is important to arrange the follow-up on these items discussed. Is additional information needed? If so, who will obtain that? Should a small group within the
Department be charged to come forth with a thoughtful proposal?
If so, who should be on that group, what is the charge, with whom
are they to meet to get outside information, and what is the timeline
for reporting back to the Chair? This information needs to come
to the Chair before the next meeting of the entire Department for
Chair input and advice regarding the possible need for further
facts before being brought to the next Department meeting.

Very importantly, when the Chair delegates responsibility, this
implies some authority and demands accountability to the Chair.

These items for discussion should be discussed calmly as faculty
recognize that no decision is to be made at this meeting, and
they have opportunity for input.

Over time with sequential meetings and discussions, the Chair
can espouse core values and Departmental tone, mission, and
consistency of purpose.

c) **Items for decision**: Most of these items will be follow-ups from
prior meetings' items that were the topics discussed, reports back
from small groups (or individuals) to obtain more information,
etc. Unlike items for discussion, which by design are to get faculty
input and to obtain additional information as needed, these items
are "the rubber hits the road." These items require decision—yes/
no, specific course of action, etc. Only occasionally should the
result of these decision items be "we need more information." If
the fact-finding group or individual has been effective and the
Chair been astute when receiving the report prior to taking this
report/recommendation to the entire Department, hopefully the
need for additional information will be limited to those situations

where suddenly new, relevant facts have emerged. *Avoid paralysis by analysis!*

> *"Action is eloquence."*
> —WILLIAM SHAKESPEARE

d) **Next implementation steps in follow-ups to any of preceding agenda items, be those items for discussiion or items for action**—Some examples are:

   i) What will the Chair specifically do in the follow-up to this meeting, prior to next meeting?

   ii) If one or more faculty members, or a small fact-finding group, have tasks to implement following the items for information, or items for discussion, the Chair should let those individuals know his/her expectations on what the deliverable is to be, and what the timeline is for this to be accomplished with notification to the Chair. Depending on the situation, the Chair may need to meet with the specific faculty member or the small group in order to flesh out the objectives and purposes, and facilitate contacts with those outside the Department, etc.

   iii) For the items with action decided, who is to do what, with what timeline, and with what deliverable

   iv) Invite Department members to bring up items they'd like considered for upcoming meetings.

8) Some general guidelines are recommended on how to run any meeting. These items below are generalized, not limited to meetings within the Department. These points below are most relevant to special one-time meetings but can apply as well to regularly scheduled sequential meetings.

a) Depending on your level of responsibility within the overall AHC, the meeting may be with:

   i) All the faculty in the Department, per the comments under listed under "7"

   ii) The Division chiefs (large Department)

   iii) The Chair/Director leadership from other Departments/Centers

   iv) Faculty from several Departments, perhaps discussing inter-Departmental team development

   v) Some/all of the other Chairs/Center Directors

b) To minimize the "pain" of any meeting:

   i) Conveniently located room of proper size, large enough so as not to be crowded, small enough that the group is not dwarfed by the expanse of empty space

   ii) Table of appropriate size around which individuals meet—facilitates direct dialogue and eye-to-eye contact

   iii) Avoid "layers of attendees," some at the table, others in the back row who thus might feel left out and not be engaged in the meeting

   iv) Avoid the "throne" complex; the Chair sits at the head of the table, but in the same size chair and at the same elevation as all attendees

   v) If a large meeting in large room, be certain of good acoustics

   vi) Start and end on time

   vii) Scheduling at convenient time

   viii) Respect opinions and input of attendees

ix) Utilize the "for information," "for discussion," "for decision," and "for follow up" agenda to keep meeting focused, productive, and "crisp."

c) For any meeting, especially for "items for discussion" and for "items for decision" where open, frank, and honest discussion is very necessary, structuring and planning ahead for the meeting is so important. Below are listed some ways to facilitate this careful planning prior to the actual meeting, assuming the Chair is the person responsible for the meeting:

i) The Chair should know prior to the meeting the outcome desired, and have a clear sense in mind as to the purpose or purposes of the meeting. This should be relatively simple if the leader called the meeting based upon his/her own initiative. Is this for open exchange of ideas but no decision? Is this meeting driven by a need for a decision? Does the Chair, as Chair of the meeting, have all the information needed? If not, where and from whom can this information be obtained, or would it be wise to add special consultants to the meeting (such as Office of Counsel)?

ii) If the meeting is being held at the request of the Dean or the CEO or the Hospital Director, connect with them ahead of time, so as to be absolutely certain of their charge, the outcome they wish from this meeting, and the timeline for action. Depending on the nature of the charge and how controversial the matter, the Chair might wish to discuss with the Dean and/or CEO whether or not it is best for the Dean/CEO to attend the meeting and present the charge.

9) The Chair should decide about the merits of minutes for meetings. These will usually prove to be very helpful. Concise, bulleted minutes will refresh the minds of participants at the subsequent meetings.

Minutes are also helpful for those unable to attend and for the Dean/ CEO if the meeting is held at his/her request.

Depending on the preference of the Chair, the minutes can be taken by the Chair or by a very senior staff person. The latter is preferable in most situations, to allow the Chair to fully concentrate on interacting with attendees and not be distracted. Those minutes by the staff person should be edited and approved by the Chair before any distribution.

If legal issues are involved, it is very prudent to have the consulting attorney take the minutes. These may be protected under attorney-client privileges, depending on the specific situation for which the Chair will need to defer to the attorney's advice.

10) The Chair needs to decide about the need for external consultants on items for discussion or items for decision, whether these are consultants from elsewhere in the AHC or external to the AHC. (see chapter 20) If they are to be included, be certain to bring them up to speed on all the issues and facts as the Chair understands those facts and issues. Alert these consultants both about attendees who may have strong opinions and about prior discussions with faculty on these issues. This will maximize the value of the consultants' attendance and input.

11) Premeeting planning is so important.

 a) Productive meetings do not "drift." Discussions need to be focused, and any decisions, clear and decisive. The Chair of the meeting must execute proper preparation, construct a wise agenda, and know the position most likely to be taken by all those in attendance. The meeting discussions should hold no surprises for the Chair. Good meeting leadership should result in the desired outcome of the meeting.

b) For any meeting anticipated to be contentious, the Chair might be well-advised:

   i) To meet ahead of time with key individuals who will be at the meeting to be certain to know "where they are coming from" on central issues

   ii) Prior to the meeting the Chair should connect with those who will be helpful and supportive

   iii) The Chair should clearly understand the issue(s) that may be contentious flash point(s) and similarly understand those issues that may be unifying at the upcoming meeting.

12) Know the people who are attending the meeting. By this is meant, "What makes them tick?" There seems to be certain definite "people styles" that emerge at meetings (see chapter 19). Remember body language and tone of voice may be more indicative of a participant's opinion than the words spoken. To run a smooth meeting, the Chair will need a certain approach to encourage or diffuse the various speakers. This Chair should know prior to the meeting the style of each attendee and if not, be perceptive enough to quickly discern this. Some of these types of behavior that may emerge and strategies to keep these individuals as part of a productive meeting are:

   a) Quiet, thoughtful: These people are often "deep thinkers," and may tend to keep thoughts to themselves. There will be times when the Chair is well-advised to meet with these people ahead of time, and if an individual's thoughts and ideas align with the desired goals of the meeting, alert him/her to expect to be called upon during the meeting for his/her thoughts and opinions. The reasons for this center on the fact that ideally the leader of the meeting should try to serve as moderator, rather than a proponent, in so far as this is possible. This heads-up to this quiet faculty member gives the person a chance to get his/her thoughts organized to respond when called upon, and if he/she is shy, will avoid embarrassing him/her.

b) Forceful, direct, dogmatic: These people have no trouble speaking up. They can be intimidating, may pontificate their ideas, and may inflame others or squelch discussion by confrontation. Even if the Chair agrees with this speaker's opinion, discussion by others is still important. The meeting leader can control the situation by thanking the speaker, acknowledging and summarizing his/her comments, and then asking to hear the opinions of other faculty and attendees. One phrasing the author has found helpful is, "Thank you for stating your thoughts so clearly. What I've heard you say is 'XXXXXX.' Now I would also like to hear what others are thinking about the issues."

c) Verbose repetitive talker: These people tend to be the ones who "think out loud." They may talk in circles, and as they convince themselves of the merits of their thoughts, they often say the same thing over and over again, although perhaps in different words. As the moderator/leader, the Chair may well need to interrupt as they "lap around the track again." Helpful wording may be, "Let me summarize your point(s) as 'YYYYY.' Did I understand you correctly? Let's now move along for the thoughts of others as well."

d) Circuitous thinker: These people usually "just don't get it." Unlike the repetitive talker who thinks out loud but is usually circling around the core issues, these circuitous thinkers are off chasing issue "A" and solution "B," when the problem is actually "P" with solution choices "Q" or "R." Again, as the moderator and leader, the Chair should acknowledge their idea(s), but bring the discussion back on target by saying something such as, "Thank you, NAME, for your assessment. I am more concerned about

'P' and our possible solutions, and let's hear what others think about 'P.'"

e) Manipulator/charmer: These faculty are the most troublesome, usually very clever, and can be subtly disruptive to the mission. All topics and discussions are seen through their frame of reference, which subconsciously (or often consciously) is, "What's in this for me? How can I turn this to my advantage?" This advantage might be "more money for me, or more lab space for me, or sow dissension in this meeting and in the Department. How can I be disruptive but mask it with my charm, undercut the leader to discredit him/her so maybe I can get that position, etc." After the meeting, these individuals push their dangerous mission by pitting one person against the other, and by innuendo around the coffeepot, in the whisper/whisper hallway conversation, etc. These individuals cannot be made part of any meaningful solution. The leader is in a tough position. If the leader acknowledges what this person has said, it gives that person credibility; if the leader disagrees and states the factual reasons, it may well give this person ammunition to use in the subsequent whisper-rumor campaign in corridor conversations. The author often found this short and pointed statement to be helpful: "You've expressed your thoughts. We need to move on to others." Once detected, these faculty are best marginalized by not including them in such meetings or decision making. These individuals will ideally find a position in another institution, perhaps with "encouragement" (see chapter 28 for how to deal with this situation, especially if essential research, clinical, or educational skills are involved, and also to avoid legal and human resource issues).

f) Always negative, nothing is "right": These are the "Gloomy Guses" of the world. They are never so happy as when they are miserable with something about which to complain. Everything is dark, and the world is out to get them or take away what they have. That said, they may have valuable insights, although from a different perspective, and in fact may be excellent clinicians and/or teachers and/or researchers. The leader can keep them involved by sayings such as, "Thank you. Very interesting. My understanding of what you said is 'SSS.' We need to be aware of that, but let's move on to other faculty's ideas on this."

13) The Chair running a meeting, during the meeting, should:

a) Be pleasant—both in words and body language

b) Be certain everyone knows everyone—especially important if there are external consultants present

c) Announce if there will be minutes and who will be taking those

d) Introduce the agenda and the purpose of the meeting and the outcome desired, such as:

   i) "We need to discuss 'a, b, and c' and decide what further information is needed and how to get that information."

   ii) "The Dean has requested we provide a list of pros and cons for 'x course of action' for his/her consideration."

   iii) "We need to review the Departmental revenues, hear from the accountant, and agree on the salary incentives as proposed by our intra-Departmental finance committee."

e) Stay calm, no matter how outrageous someone's comment(s)

f) Have boundaries of professional communication that are clear to all in attendance

g) Be factual

h) Have no "you messages"; these are the accusatory or belittling directives at one or more attendees, which almost always will create defensive postures and can poison the meeting with tension. Examples of what to avoid might be, "I cannot understand how YOU could have said that," or "YOU just don't understand," or "How could YOU have done that!"

i) Utilize an appropriate sense of humor. (Most historians agree that Abraham Lincoln was a master of this use of humor. Doris Kearns's book *Team of Rivals* has many examples of this.) Humor needs to be skillfully utilized at the proper moment. This humor:

    1) Helps keep participants alert

    2) Is extremely helpful to diffuse tension

    3) Does not mean telling a joke, but more often is a play on words

    4) Must be clean

    5) Never belittles or demeans others with humor, but it is perfectly OK for the Chair to poke fun at him/herself

    6) Is very valuable in getting discussion "back on track"

14) Follow-up after the meeting is extremely important.

  a) If this was a single stand-alone meeting, the Chair should:

    i) Follow up to implement decisions made

    ii) Brief Senior Leadership on results, if appropriate, which is mandatory if the meeting was held and conducted at their request

  b) If this meeting is one in a series of meetings, the Chair should:

    i) Be certain to follow up on all matters discussed and decided

    ii) Meet (or connect by phone or e-mail as appropriate) with any newly assigned subgroup(s) or individual(s) to review their charge, confirm steps and timelines, and reaffirm the deliverables

iii) If this was a meeting where subgroups and/or individuals made reports, thank them.

c) Remember, if the Chair delegates responsibility, he/she should also extend authority and insist upon specific and timely accountability.

> *"Make everything as simple as possible, but not simpler."*
> —ALBERT EINSTEIN

Be a Leader
Make a Difference
Enjoy!

CHAPTER 24

Strategies for Collaborative Win-Win Negotiations, Difficult Conversations, and Conflict Resolution

> *"He [She] that handles a matter wisely shall find good."*
>
> —FROM PROVERBS 16:20, KING JAMES VERSION

> *"Timing has a lot to do with the outcome of a rain dance."*
>
> —AUTHOR UNKNOWN

> *"Successful people are always looking for opportunities to help others. Unsuccessful people are always asking, 'What's in it for me?'"*
>
> —BRIAN TRACY

In approaching any situation or setting where issues need resolution, there are helpful overall concepts that the Chair should keep in mind.

Faculty, like all people, will respond to positive reinforcement. Money/ salary is less of a motivator. If incentivized by money alone, people will do what they are paid to do, and no more. If something else occurs that needs attention, time, and effort and it is not in the payment line, it

LEADING DEPARTMENT EXCELLENCE

won't get done. One the other hand, if the salary is based on performance with positive reinforcement, acknowledgement, and praise, the individual will usually respond to the challenge of the new, unexpected event and act. This concept should be carried forward by the Chair to the conversations and negotiations that are detailed next.

In summary of what is to follow, there are **some key strategic concepts and efforts that the Chair needs to do prior: a) to negotiating, b) to a difficult conversation, or c) to seeking conflict resolution.** These are:

1) Preparation and/or individual conversation with those involved prior to any meeting

2) Know the positive and negative consequences for those involved should discussions succeed or fail

3) Have as many objective relevant facts as is realistic

4) Attempt to understand or at least predict everyone's "why"

5) Know all the areas involved so as to be able to broaden the topic(s) to be discussed, or conversely to focus the conversations

6) Seek common ground and then steer the conversations to focus on positive solutions

> *"Words that soak into your ears are whispered...not yelled."*
> —Author unknown

As a general guideline for conversations to mentor future improved performance or actions, here are some helpful steps:

1) The Chair should ask the person, "What did you do well?" followed by "Why did you do it that way?"

2) The Chair may then tell the person what the Chair thought was done well and why he/she thought it was done well.

3) The Chair should then ask, "What do you think you could have done differently?" followed by "Why do you think you should have done it differently?"

4) The Chair should then follow with what he/she thinks the individual should have done differently and why that would have been a better way.

5) Hopefully then this above conversation will foster the ensuing productive dialogue on future situations, responsibilities, and expectations in deliverables and accountability.

> *"In order to win a man [woman] to your cause, you must first reach his [her] heart, the high road to his [her] reason."*
>
> —ABRAHAM LINCOLN

In negotiations a productive approach is to consider this as the coming together of two or more individuals (or groups) to discuss issues, choices, or challenges and then to agree to conclusions, solutions, and/or courses of action acceptable to all. This cannot be "I win, you lose"; for with time, the "win-lose" will become "lose-lose." This is a very broad definition, applicable to many settings.

There are many negotiating scenarios: a few examples of those that might involve the Chair are:

- Meeting with one or more faculty in the Department to decide on a system to allocate support resources, be that operating room time, clinical time, laboratory bench space, or office space

- Meeting with the Dean over hard-money issues

- Series of meetings to increase the AHC resource allocation to the Department, such as a special operating room designated for trauma, more laboratory space to accommodate increases in NIH-funded research, more support from development/ advancement for philanthropy, or the new construction of an off-site clinical building and/or surgical center

- Meetings with Senior Leadership for support of increase in salary for some of the faculty in the Department who have assumed major administrative roles in the AHC (such as revisions in the medical school curriculum, administration of graduate education, administrative role in clinical practice plans, assistant or associate dean responsibilities, etc.)

Prior to the meeting, the Chair entering into a negotiation is well-advised to learn the following:

1) The general background of the individual(s) with whom the Chair is negotiating; this is the type of information on the CV or on the AHC website

2) The relevant other and more-detailed information about the individual with whom he/she is negotiating as it pertains to the specific current discussion or negotiation, and what might be of particular interest, value, or concern to this individual on the topic(s) for discussion and negotiation

3) Are there other big items "on the plates" of the people with whom the Chair is negotiating? For example, if the Chair is seeking additional funding or resource allocation, the other demands at the AHC for those same resources may have a major impact on the flexibility with which the other party will approach discussions. Are there other creative sources of funding or combining of programs to make more efficient use of funding that is available?

STRATEGIES FOR COLLABORATIVE WIN-WIN...

4) The Chair should be crystal clear in his/her mind as to the needs of the Department. The "need(s)" are defined as what is required to improve the situation, *not* what is needed as a minimum to survive.

5) The Chair must know his/her Best Alternative to a Negotiated Agreement (BATNA) (9). Anyone getting into these dialogues has to know those core items/issues that must be maintained and cannot be compromised/sacrificed. In other words, the Chair must know the strengths of his/her prenegotiation situation, such that the status quo (i.e., the failure of the negotiation) is a better alternative than accepting the negotiated settlement proposed by the other party. From prior research on the other individuals' situations and goals, the Chair should try to deduce the BATNA of the others in the meeting. The Chair had best know and understand where the edge of the cliff is in brinkmanship.

6) The Chair needs to know what possible alternatives might be available or be created, to build upon and improve the BATNA and that will not require a total restart of negotiations. In other words, the Chair prior to the negotiations should have a backup plan that is viable and beneficial should negotiations fail initially. This reserve parachute will avoid the need to agree to something that is of no benefit.

7) The Chair should know what the other person's/people's needs might be with which the Chair might be able to help. Thus, the Chair will hopefully gain what he/she needs at the same time as helping the other people with their situation.

8) Structure the setting, time, and amenities (coffee, tea, cheese, etc.) of the meeting to foster a collaborative, relaxed, nonconfrontational atmosphere.

9) If possible prior to the meeting, the Chair should have ideas to bring to the discussions where the Chair's goals and needs are similar or have common threads with those of the other people. This will

establish a pattern of win-win early in the meeting where agreements are achieved on steps and solutions that benefit all involved.

In the actual meeting, the Chair should:

1) Try to frame the big picture within a resultant win-win framework of common ground and goals.

2) Remember the KISS principle of "Keep It Simple Stupid," and try not to get bogged down in details until there is agreement on fifty-thousand-foot, big-picture perspectives. Once that is accomplished, the sandbox is defined with a big-picture win-win scenario, making it easier to sort out and agree on some of the lesser items that are necessary for the bigger goal.

3) Then move on to other issues where agreement will be more difficult to achieve.

4) Be creative using ideas from others as well as the Chair's for solutions that align incentives, improve the situation for all involved in the negotiations, and are fair to all concerned.

5) Be observant of body language of the others in the room. This yields valuable information as to what is making sense to or is comfortable for the other person vs. what is perceived by him/her to be threatening or unacceptable.

> *"Do not corner something that you know is meaner than you."*
> —Author unknown

6) Avoid brinkmanship. It may be tempting to "be macho," to issue edicts, and to threaten to walk away. Unless the Chair holds a huge asset advantage such that the others have no choice but to acquiesce, the risk is that the bluff will be called, and the Chair will either walk

away with far less than needed and/or have to come "crawling back to the table" with real loss of bargaining position and strength.

7) When involving finances, business activities, and/or resource re-allocations, have a business plan, including return on investment outcomes (i.e., a business plan proposal with financial and/or legal analysis). This plan should include an assessment of "does everyone benefit, or do some benefit and some lose?"

> *"Never allow a person to tell you no who doesn't have the power to say yes."*
> —ELEANOR ROOSEVELT

8) If the negotiations seem to be at a standstill once under way, the Chair needs to be alert that this may be a tactic used by the others to entice a "cave-in"; or it may be that matters indeed are at an impasse. The more that the Chair knows about the other individual's situation, motives, and BATNA, the easier it is for the Chair to make the distinctions and decisions.

9) If there is a legitimate impasse, one very helpful technique is to introduce some additional information and insights that broaden—or alternatively, focus—the dialogue by reframing the discussions. In other words, change the sandbox, reset the discussion, and open up new opportunities and avenues for productive discussions.

10) Remember, decisions can always be deferred, for "further information and further thought." Once decisions are made, especially at the institutional level, it may be difficult to go back and rework them.

11) In negotiations, never make a decision under duress.

12) Tone and style of all involved are keys to success for a win-win. Approach the negotiations with integrity, good intentions, humility, and legitimate purpose—and an appropriate sense of humor—and

if the counterparts have the same style, the chances for a successful win-win are greatly enhanced.

13) If those individuals with whom the Chair is negotiating are arrogant, scheming, and dogmatic, the chances of success are much less certain and much more difficult; the possibility of success will improve significantly if both parties:

a) Sincerely listen to what the others say and listen to understand, and thoughtfully consider what the others say

b) If disagreeing with what has been stated, focus on the big picture and the positives being sought and calmly make the counterpoints based on facts.

c) Stick with facts, not emotional statements. For example, "I hear what you say. You make the point that XXXXX. But we have some other facts to consider, namely QQQQ. We agree on YYYYYY, and ZZZZZZ are relevant and we should fold those facts into our discussions."

d) If someone gets emotional and starts "ventilating," don't let him/her derail the entire effort. After an appropriate but not too lengthy time, gently steer the discussion back to "cool calm facts." Responding emotionally to emotion is counterproductive.

e) Always separate the person from the message. The sincere attitude of "I really do not like your idea for ZZZZ facts, but I like and respect you" is key to remember in these situations.

f) Welcome people who have new, constructive factual ideas that are relevant.

g) How and when to provide feedback to listening is important. Do not interrupt. Acknowledge with respect what has been stated and heard. Positions should be stated factually and with conviction, but not with emotion.

h) Flexibility is *not* the same as indecision and does not mean yielding. In fact, often with flexibility by all involved, new and creative ideas and solutions will arise centered on areas of common interest, which benefit all in a win-win result.

i) When matters get tense, or someone has been emotional, humor is a powerfully useful tool. Please see chapters 19 and 21 for comments on appropriate use of humor. In brief, the Chair should keep it clean, never belittling unless to poke fun at him/herself. Ideally the humor will have an appropriate message. Abraham Lincoln was a master at this, as was Ronald Reagan.

> *"I have wondered at times about what the Ten Commandments would have looked like if Moses had run them through the US Congress."*
>
> —Ronald Reagan

> *"I've laid down the law, though, to everyone from now on about anything that happens: no matter what time it is, wake me, even if it's in the middle of a Cabinet meeting."*
>
> —Ronald Reagan

Difficult conversations require many of the same style strengths and disciplines as negotiation. However, for the Chair these conversations usually do not involve negotiating an outcome. In these conversations there is usually a power figure and an individual of less authority or rank, with the power figure delivering an unwanted and often surprisingly unpleasant and unexpected message. These conversations most often involve one of two scenarios.

1) In the most common situation, **the Chair is the power figure** and is forced to discipline or even to fire a faculty member or resident

or fellow or staff person (see chapter 28). Note that for faculty, for residents and fellows, and for staff, the contemporaneous on-going documentation of the offenses, attempted remediation, mentoring, and sequential meetings is essential. These meetings for difficult conversations should always be attended by an impartial and appropriate third individual. If the person being disciplined or fired is a female or URM, so also should be this impartial third individual. In all situations, the purpose for this third person is "the second set of ears as a witness," to avoid subsequent difficulties should the aggrieved party mistake what was discussed or challenge what was said at the meeting. Ideally, this third individual will be someone of authority in the Department and at the same time has a legitimate reason to be included because of the subject(s) being discussed--such as an Associate Chair, the residency Program Director, or the senior Program Administrator. This third individual should not be legal counsel, as this will prompt the other individual to seek legal recourse. That said, input from legal counsel to the Chair is essential prior to these meetings.

The author has found it extremely valuable to actually role-play the conversation with someone from the Office of Counsel ahead of time; this goes a long way to avoid inappropriate or unwise comments by the Chair. The Chair's position embodies honesty, sincerity, and calmness. The Chair will be direct, factual, firm, and unemotional.

2) In the second, and hopefully rare scenario, the Chair is being disciplined or relieved of his/her administrative position as Chair. In this setting **the Dean or CEO is certainly the power figure**.

If the situation is one of discipline of the Chair, he/she is advised to seek clear explanation with details of the problem(s), changes, and/or actions the Dean wishes the Chair to initiate, the timeline for those, and the outcome desired.

If the Chair is being dismissed, the Chair must remember that administrative positions are at the pleasure of Senior Leadership. Although the academic appointment may be with tenure, the administrative appointment as Chair is not. That said, hopefully cordial, productive discussion may follow as to a possible future role the resigning Chair may occupy in the AHC—be it teaching, research, or patient care. It is unusual for the Senior Leadership to request the Chair to leave the AHC, as most Chairs will have academic tenure. If tenure is to be severed, this will usually involve the Office of Counsel for the AHC, attorneys for the Chair, and some sort of tenure buyout.

Conflict resolution with the Chair mediating between two or more individuals poses a complex combination of negotiating and difficult conversations. The similarities of skill sets required match those of negotiation, for the Chair is mediating and negotiating to find common ground between the two parties who are in "combat mode." These skills and steps are detailed earlier in this chapter. The similarity with the difficult conversations is the "heat" of hostility and accusations between the antagonists. In these conflict resolution scenarios, the Chair will need to move smoothly and skillfully to and fro between the parties, attempting to identify common grounds shared by the conflicting individuals as would be done with negotiating. At the same time, the Chair will need to utilize the authority position to enforce a calm, disciplined, factual discussion that moves from irrational conflict to areas of common agreement. At this point, the negotiating skills come to the fore as the Chair moves the parties to build on areas of agreement.

Be a Leader
Make a Difference
Enjoy!

CHAPTER 25

Confidential Information—
Definitions, Types, and Challenges

"Lettin' the cat outta the bag is a whole lot easier than puttin' it back in."

—AUTHOR UNKNOWN

The more facts a Chair has, the more effective that Chair will be. Some information is common knowledge, out there for all who are attentive to gather; some information is privileged, and must be kept in confidence. It is essential to know the difference.

If the Chair has a reputation for being trustworthy, honest, and discreet, other Chairs or faculty at the AHC who are seeking advice, or just want to "ventilate frustrations," will confide in the Chair. This Chair's reputation is to be treasured and not taken for granted. One betrayal will ruin that reputation; it can never be retrieved.

Privacy issues are so important. In addition to faculty in the Department or other Chairs as referenced above, Senior Leadership may seek advice from those they trust. Of necessity, Senior Leadership will have information and/or be pondering decisions that need to remain confidential during deliberations until Senior Leadership deems it prudent to distribute the information, implement the decision, or abandon the planned effort. At times, one or a small group of Chairs will be asked to meet with Senior Leadership to provide information, and Senior Leadership may well seek his/her/their opinion. That confidence must never be betrayed by that/those Chair(s).

Examples of such privileged situations are:

1) Interfacing with Senior Leadership:

   a) The Chair is on a leadership task force commissioned by Senior Leadership to produce recommendations to solve a challenging and/or controversial issue with a report that is to be confidential. The appropriate behavior never breaks that confidence.

   b) One of the Senior Leaders comes to the Chair, out of respect for the person and the insights, to "float a trial balloon" for an idea the Senior Leader has had. He/she wants to think-tank with this selected Chair.

   c) The Chair is on a standing committee that meets with Senior Leadership to discuss possible future planning issues.

2) Interfacing with co-Chair(s):

   a) Another Chair comes to this Chair, knowing that this Chair has solved a tough issue in his/her Department, and is now confronting an analogous situation and wants advice—what to do, whom to contact, possible courses of action, pitfalls?

   b) Another Chair is confronting a very difficult family situation and is not so much looking for advice as for an opportunity to talk, knowing the very personal information will go no further.

3) Interfaces with faculty in the Chair's Department or at times, even in another Department:

   a) These are often personal situations, such as family difficulties or financial problems.

   b) Professional issues may include career-trajectory advice, research or clinical difficulties, being recruited to another AHC, challenges posed by PhD candidates/residents/other faculty, etc.

4) Conversations initiated by staff members whose issues often center on HR situations, harassment, etc., or like faculty may have personal family issues

There are some key exceptions when confidentiality may not be possible. These scenarios usually involve issues such as violence, threatened violence, possible suicide concerns, sexual harassment allegations, etc. Before breaching confidentiality, it is best to first seek the advice of in-house Office of Counsel and/or the Dean on how best to proceed.

Be a Leader
Make a Difference
Enjoy!

C. Faculty Challenges

CHAPTER 26

Successful Recruiting of Excellent and Diverse Faculty, and The Important Role of the Offer Letter

> *"Your task is not to foresee the future, but to enable it."*
>
> —ANTOINE DE SAINT-EXUPERY

> *"A leader needs a true heart, a strong mind, and a great deal of courage."*
>
> —HARRY TRUMAN

Excellent faculty are the absolute core value of any successful academic Department/Center. Excellence should be sought and nurtured with energy and diligence. This task is one of the most important responsibilities of the Chair, and it will be one of the most significant long-lasting impacts and legacies of the Chair.

What features should the leader seek in new faculty, whether that individual comes from within the trainee ranks or from outside the AHC? These traits are much easier to ascertain when recruiting from within. That said, due diligence is essential to attempt the acquisition of reliable objective information on external candidates, and this is difficult.

What comprises the excellent faculty member whom the Chair is seeking? Research brilliance or clinical acumen is not enough. The following are some, but not all, of the qualities that an excellent faculty candidate should possess:

1) Already has, or if early in career, has the potential ability to master three of the five supporting legs of the academic stool; those skill sets are research, teaching, clinical skills, community outreach, and administration

2) Talent as a team player. This is a key personality trait, difficult to mentor or teach and has several facets:

   a) Espouses the viewpoint that a rising tide floats all boats, so "my successes reflect well on the Department and therefore help my cofaculty"; similarly with genuine enthusiasm he/she will value the successes of others in the Department, recognizing that: "The accomplishments of my cofaculty benefit me as well."

   b) Avoiding the behavior of: "What's mine is mine, and what's yours is mine." This is very dangerous and destructive for all the cofaculty and often also for the individual perpetrator.

   c) Mutual respect such that the researcher respects and values the clinician, and the clinician likewise regards highly and appreciates the researcher; each genuinely acknowledges the validity and value of the other's contributions to the whole mission. By appreciating and admiring the contributions of others, each faculty member can take pride in his/her accomplishments without arrogance.

   d) All faculty members, whether in research, clinical care, or education, appreciate the value of administrative effort and of community outreach activities.

3) Has a positive attitude: this does not mean the faculty member has to think like the Pollyanna for whom "everything is lovely and perfect;"

however, it is important to see the glass as half-full, not half-empty. These faculty appreciate the positives and will help the leaders seek imaginative and constructive solutions for the negatives.

4) Integrity is so important. Without this, all of the other attributes have little value.

5) Is willing to cheerfully work hard and efficiently. This has always been important and now is progressively essential in the evolving era of decreasing external funding for research and for clinical activities. The hours of effort are not enough by themselves, for the faculty member must be creatively and productively efficient with time and institutional resources, be those resources space, finances, and/or staff support.

6) Has a genuine desire to contribute to the field of his/her expertise, and to improve the understanding, treatment, education/teaching of the diseases and disorders in that area of health—by research, clinical care, or both. These candidates come to the AHC for "the right reasons."

The Chair is central to the recruiting process. The existing faculty and spouses/partners are key allies in this endeavor. If the Chair has a reputation for fairness, integrity, vision, hard work, and team-building, the faculty will be enthusiastic and positive in their interactions with the potential new faculty member. The opposite is death to recruiting; unhappy faculty who express dissatisfaction will put a screeching brake on the possibility for excellent new faculty recruiting. The same holds true for Departmental spouses' or partners' interactions with the recruit's counterpart.

> *"Everyone wants to live on top of the mountain, but all the happiness and growth occurs while you're climbing it."*
> —ANDY ROONEY

There are several important questions to ask before initiating the recruiting processes. Is this faculty candidate to be from within the AHC, from another AHC, and with or without a formal national search? Is the Department seeking to fill a junior, midcareer, or senior-career position? What combination of research, clinical, and educational skill sets does the Department need to augment? What resources are available? What are the sources for those resource assets of space, money, time, support staff, etc.? Which faculty should be involved in the search? Are there members of the Department who still need to be convinced about the need for this new recruit? Are there faculty in other Departments with whom the recruit would be working or interfacing, who should therefore also be involved in the recruitment process? What should be in the offer letter to the potential new faculty member?

1) **Recruiting of new junior faculty from within your AHC** will come from the ranks of trainees. There are many scenarios, each with pros and/or cons. Depending on the promotion systems at the AHC, the appointment may be as Instructor, Senior Instructor, or Assistant Professor. In each of these scenarios, the Chair and/or the faculty will have personal knowledge of the potential faculty member's individual strengths, weaknesses, and most probable career trajectory. The sources of these internal junior recruits are:

   a) Residents from the same AHC, directly from the residency training

   b) Successful PhD graduates from the Departmental PhD programs

   c) Residents who have remained to take a post-residency subspecialty fellowship at the AHC

   d) Residents who take subspecialty fellowships at another AHC and might want to return

   e) Former PhD students who have taken postdoctoral appointments at another AHC and might wish to return

f) Residents from elsewhere who take fellowships at the AHC and who are being considered for faculty positions

g) Postdoctoral appointees at the AHC being considered for a faculty appointment

2) The names of **potential recruits from "outside" the AHC** come from word-of-mouth information, candidates' responses to the Department's efforts from a national search, candidates who have initiated the contact based on their desire to relocate to the geographic area, or because of the AHC's/Department's strong reputation.

3) There are **several issues that must be considered in this recruiting of junior faculty**, whether the recruiting process is focused on internal and/or external candidates:

a) The necessity to comply with state and federal regulations/laws on the diversity factors of race/gender/sexuality. This compliance is an area of ever-increasing complexity, and the new leader will need input from in-house HR and especially the Office of Counsel on what is legally mandated. For example, to satisfy diversity pool legal obligations as it applies to internal candidates, and if new faculty are to be selected from residents and/or fellows already in the Department as graduating trainees, how is the candidate pool defined?

   i) Is the diversity pool defined as limited to those residents and fellows in place after selection for those positions?

   ii) Or are the diversity pool size and breadth criteria satisfied with the much larger applicant pool from which those residents/fellows were selected in the prior years, based on the fact that candidates for residency and especially fellowships are screened as trainees with faculty potential?

b) Prior accurate and objective assessment of the Department needs, and how those needs meld with the needs and visions of the AHC as a whole in times of decreasing resources

c) Accurate financial projections of budgets and funding sources for start-up packages

d) Approval requirements from the Office of the Dean and the Office of Finance, as may be mandated at that AHC

e) Agreement within the current Departmental and/or Divisional faculty for the need of a new faculty member and the skill sets and career trajectory that is the best "fit" for the Departmental needs; ideally this agreement will be a consensus, but on occasion when there is strong agreement but not consensus, the Chair will need to mentor the dissenter with the goal of convincing him/her with facts and logic and vision.

f) Junior faculty recruits will often be less expensive for resources than more senior recruits, especially in clinical areas. For research faculty, the financial analysis may be more complex if the more senior faculty bring with them current grants that offset their salary and contribute to indirect costs; also the midcareer research faculty will be more of a known quantity in terms of predicting future successes with grant funding.

g) These new faculty, if junior, will not bring with them any national reputation, established clinical programs, or national research grant funding.

4) **Important general considerations for each academic level of recruitment:**

a) Evaluation with due diligence is more difficult for external junior faculty candidates than for potential junior faculty from within the AHC. The Departmental leaders will have personal insights from direct contact with the internal potential faculty candidate and have a "feel" for the likely career trajectory. It will be hard to predict the trajectory of the external junior candidate, as the career is so embryonic, and the candidate is not personally known.

b) Midcareer faculty:

i) How to define "midcareer"?

(1) Age? This is not that helpful. Some younger individuals have amazing career accomplishments, not just potential, and are competitive with older faculty in their academic successes. Does this individual combine the personal accomplishments with the team spirit of helping others toward a common vision? There is one cautionary consideration. Does this person's fire in the belly and early extraordinary accomplishments come at the price of not being a team player? Is this a self-centered achiever who runs roughshod over others in the pursuit of personal success?

(2) Accomplishments to date are more important than age, for it is not the number of heartbeats that count for academic promotion.

(3) Anticipated further career potential is noteworthy but must be based upon solid evidence, not just hope. Beware of "smoke and mirrors."

ii) New midcareer faculty can be promoted from within from the junior faculty or can be recruited from outside.

iii) Why is the Department considering expanding the number of midcareer faculty from outside? If the Department has

220

wisely selected junior faculty in years past, and if there is a good mentoring program in place, should not the internal pool for promotion to midcareer rank preclude the need for outside recruits to this rank? If this is not the situation, the Chair might need to focus on how junior faculty are selected and mentored, and the opportunities for improvement in those processes.

c) Senior faculty:

i) As for midcareer faculty, these senior appointments can come by promotion from within or from another AHC.

ii) If an external recruit, why is this being done? Is this for divisional leadership? Is this to initiate a new area of expertise within the Department? If not one of those situations, what is being sought that has been not "grown in-house"? The reasoning and need for introspection here is the same as for midcareer faculty.

iii) If this is an external recruit, it is key to know, "Why does this person want to move his/her established career at this senior point in accomplishments?" Are there burned bridges where he/she was? Does he/she have excess baggage? Is he/she burned out and now wants to coast? Is this individual truly outstanding and now seeks new opportunity? Did this person get overlooked to be Chair at the current AHC and now wants to move, and once settled in the new AHC, then compete for the Chair position by undermining current leadership?

iv) External recruits will have the potential value of "fresh blood and ideas" but will carry the risk that the new AHC won't know "the location and size of the warts."

> *"There are risks and costs to action. But they are far less than the long-range risks of comfortable inaction."*
>
> —John F. Kennedy

The recruiting visits to the Department and AHC need to be thoughtfully and prudently organized. In these processes, the internal faculty candidates should be accorded the same courtesies as the external candidates for that same academic rank and position.

1) First visit, assuming the internal candidate as well as the external candidates have had some preliminary vetting:

   a) Interviews with Chair, key Departmental leadership, and faculty with whom the candidate will interface

   b) Exit interview with Chair

   c) Follow-up by the Chair after the first visit:

      i) Chair discussions with other interviewers for their feedback

      ii) Appropriate phone calls by the Chair for insightful specific due-diligence purposes from those who know the faculty candidate, and learn if each would, if asked, be able to provide a strong reference letter

      iii) Phone call to candidate for dialogue, which can range all the way from "Great first visit from everyone's perspective and let's plan your next visit!" to "Unfortunately the Department (or the candidate) does not think this is a good fit."

      iv) If there is to be a second visit, the Chair and candidate need to discuss the purpose(s) of the visit and with whom the candidate will meet. Also, if the candidate is a midcareer or established-career candidate—or if for a research position—

the candidate may be requested to make an academic presentation

2) Second visit:

a) Interview with Chair

b) Interviews with key Departmental faculty who missed the first visit

c) Interviews with key faculty in other Departments with whom this candidate will interface and collaborate should he/she join the AHC faculty

d) For more senior-faculty recruits, especially if institutional resources are to be involved, interviews with Dean, Hospital Director (if a recruit who will have clinical responsibilities), and other Senior Leadership as appropriate and consistent with that AHC's policies at this rank

e) Often on the second visit, the spouse, significant other, or partner may also visit. This individual should be given a tour of the city and residential area, and be given child care and school information if relevant, especially if there are children involved with special needs.

f) Social dinner with candidate and spouse, significant other, or partner with appropriate persons from Department

g) The Chair should get immediate feedback from all the other interviewers to learn of their support or their concerns

h) Exit interview with Chair, at which time (assuming excellent feedback) there should be rather detailed and specific discussions in anticipation of what might be in the offer letter if the visit has gone well. The Chair and the candidate should agree on the names for external references. If the candidate balks at any external individuals with whom the Chair has previously had discussions, the reasons should be pursued. However, if the visit has not been productive, the candidate needs to be so informed at this time.

3) Third visit, if necessary:

a) Further discussions and resolution of matters that are to be considered in the offer letter

b) Faculty candidate and spouse, partner, significant other actively pursue housing situation, and schooling issues

> *"Shallow men believe in luck or in circumstance.*
> *Strong men believe in cause and effect."*
> —RALPH WALDO EMERSON

After the due-diligence calls, with information thus gleaned now combined with information gained from the candidate visits, there are **factors for the Chair to consider** carefully about the individual faculty candidate and the Departmental/Divisional needs before making an offer. Based upon the information learned:

1) Is the type of individual being sought (see chapter 19 for discussion of faculty types) : The triple-talented researcher-clinician-educator? A solid "heavy lifter truck loader"? Clinical leader? Brilliant researcher? Master educator?

2) What is the balance expected for this new potential faculty member's effort in clinical activity, education, research, administration, and/or outreach? Do these expectations match the faculty candidate's potential?

3) Does this individual have the potential to be a future "barn burner" superstar? The potential new faculty member should have the "fire

in the belly" with focused energy, regardless of being an internal or external candidate, and regardless of the professional activity balance being sought. The Chair should be aware that it is essential to try to ascertain what motivates the "fire in the belly" and attempt to predict if this faculty candidate will be a team player who will:

a) Move the team ball forward

b) Understand the need for team interests and personal interests to be synergistic and mutually beneficial, rather than viewing himself/herself as more important than the team.

c) The faculty trait most destructive to the Department and to be avoided if at all possible is that of the individual who seeks to move his/her career forward by bringing others down, by exhibiting his/her successes while torpedoing those of peers, almost always "behind the back" and masked within a fake team allegiance.

4) The Chair if possible should select new faculty candidates who will be of value to the AHC, as well as the Department. In the coming years, with the needs for increasing productivity from the AHC in the face of decreasing resources, the potential value of any new faculty member must be assessed in terms of the AHC needs, not just those of the Department. Will this new faculty member mesh with strong faculty in other Departments in building a key "product line"? For example, in basic, translational, or clinical research are there strong collaborative opportunities across several Departments or Centers that will potentiate the successes for extramural research funding? In clinical areas, does the potential new faculty member have skills that interdigitate with clinical activity in more than one Department? Examples of these might be:

a) A new faculty member with outstanding credentials in Cardiac Anesthesia will potentiate the successes of multi-specialty Heart Program that includes faculty from multiple Departments, with great benefit to patients, to the reputation of the AHC, and to finances.

b) An Orthopaedic surgeon recruit with world-class expertise in limb salvage significantly enhances the care possibilities available to patients under the care of Surgical Oncologists or Radiation Therapists in a cancer center.

c) Thus, these types of recruits should benefit the broad visions and reputations of the entire AHC, not just those of a single Department.

5) Prestige for the AHC can be a fickle target to pursue by trying to recruit established world-class faculty from outside, whether those recruits are research or clinical experts. If they are that famous and that successful, why are they movable? Is there unknown baggage? Will the commitment of AHC and Department resources be so great as to negate the benefits of this new senior recruit? If the Department already has up-and-coming future superstars, the incremental resources might well be better spent on those in-house individuals who a) are well-known in terms of those key intangibles; and b) are hopefully already interdigitated within multiple Departments and Centers.

6) The situation of the accompanying spouse or partner is important and progressively more common with two-career couples. This individual may be in his/her own right a legitimate new AHC faculty member based on merit. That said, there are some items to assess. If the careers of the two individuals are in the same area, issues of inurement must be addressed proactively. If this accompanying individual has skill sets better suited to another portion of the University, such as an undergraduate campus faculty position, the presence or absence of tenure track position availability can be a stumbling block. If the career of this person is in schoolteaching,

law, business, etc., the AHC may have to reach out to the community at large to help identify possible career opportunities in one of these areas outside the AHC. Often contacts via trustees or other faculty spouses may be very helpful.

> *"Without ambition one starts nothing. Without work one finishes nothing. The prize will not be sent to you. You have to win it."*
> —RALPH WALDO EMERSON

Financial considerations:

1) Is this a major recruit of established talent and worth significant assets of the AHC and Department?

2) If this midcareer faculty member is promoted from within, or recruited externally, a resource package may be required, and if so the details will depend on the specifics of the case.

3) If the faculty member is junior, internal or external, often some resources will be required, although usually much less than for the preceding two scenarios.

4) Regardless of the academic rank of the recruit, where is/are source(s) of these recruitment assets? Can they be entirely borne by the Department, or will resources be required from the AHC, (hospital, medical school, faculty practice plan)—or, as is the most likely scenario, will there be a combination of these resource assets?

5) If some asset source is external to Department, is it "free" or is there a payback of those dollars to the source (i.e., the Dean and/or the hospital)? Almost always there is a payback, especially with the future resource constrictions. A business plan must be developed up

front for this payback. Will the payback come from incremental hospital reimbursements resulting from increase in hospital billings? Note that this may be problematic with emerging accountable care organization (ACO) financial models.

6) Will this recruit lead to incremental income for that Division or Department? This demands that the Chair make a realistic factual business assessment—including, but not limited to, shifts in market share in clinical activity, increased RVUs, better resulting data on pay-for-performance models, etc. In basic research, with difficulties in the NIH pay-line constrictions, and with the fact that for every dollar brought in grants, incremental institutional dollars are required, financial modeling needs to be precise—and may rely on endowment revenues as well.

7) What is the lead time before income streams occur for clinicians? Significant details are imposed by the sequential needs for state licensure, AHC institutional credentialing, malpractice liability insurance, and acceptance on third-party-payor insurance panels. There are more details on this subsequently in this chapter (see pages 233-234). What are the reimbursement mechanisms from third-party carriers? Will the clinical practice have low or high RVU potential? Will this practice have significant Medicaid or nonpay patients?

8) If research faculty, does the person already have grants? If so and an external candidate, are those grants moveable?

9) If a young research faculty recruit without grants, the letter needs to specify the expectations for securing extramural research funding, the amounts, and the timelines.

10) Are there intellectual property, technology transfer, or conflict-of-interest issues that need to be addressed proactively?

11) If the above considerations are not favorable, what are the other positives to justify the recruit?

The **essential offer letter** is exceedingly important for several reasons.

1) As a recruiting tool, this letter provides the opportunity to be certain that both the Department (and AHC) and the potential faculty member have a clear understanding of the "sandbox" and a clear documentation on all the matters as discussed during the recruitment. The properly written offer letter will document these specific items to the benefit of the AHC, the Department, the Chair, and the recruit. (See Appendix A and Appendix B.)

2) The inclusive and detailed offer letter is so very helpful for the Chair and the new recruit to use as a benchmark for the new faculty member's progress toward goals in the first years on the faculty in the Department.

3) The well-crafted initial offer letter is key for retention of faculty who subsequently meet or exceed expectations, as it will justify current and future expenditure of AHC resources and/or academic promotion (see chapter 27).

4) Equally important, and unfortunately necessary, the initial offer letter and the subsequent poor progress reports accrued in this faculty file will be key documentation to justify the Chair's decision not to retain the faculty member (see chapter 28).

5) The offer letter, although having legal status, is best written by the Chair in nonlegal language (see Appendix A and Appendix B). Once written by the Chair and before being sent to the recruited possible new faculty member, this letter should be vetted by the Office of Counsel and edited as needed for legal purposes—but this letter should be in plain-English prose, not legalese. It would seem prudent that any offer letter be signed by the Dean (or CEO/Dean), the Hospital CEO, the director of the Faculty Practice Plan (if clinical activity is expected), and the Chair of the Department (and Director of a Center, if applicable). There should be a place for the prospective

new faculty member to countersign his/her agreement and acceptance of terms.

a) It is helpful and accurate to start this letter with this suggested sentence, "On behalf of our Department and AHC, I am writing to detail the important features of all our cordial discussions relative to your joining our Department of XXXX. This letter is intended to be certain that we are including all the items that we have discussed that are mutually important." The letter can conclude with wording such as, "On behalf of the AHC and the Department, I emphasize our enthusiasm for the possibility that you will be joining our faculty. If you have any questions or wish further clarification, please let me know so that those matters can be addressed and included in our final offer letter. We have enclosed two copies of our letter. If you agree that this letter accurately indicates all the matters we've discussed and agreed upon, please cosign in the space indicated, keep one copy for yourself, and return the other to the Department Chair's office."

a) There are several elements to the best offer letter, some with some flexibility based upon negotiable items, and some items that for legal reasons are not negotiable unless cleared by both the Dean (or CEO), by the Hospital if hospital resources are involved, by the head of the Faculty Practice Plan if financial support comes from that source, and by the Office of Counsel. The custom may well vary from one AHC to another, but with today's economic challenges to AHC with various revenue sources and models, it is important for both the Chair and the faculty candidate to recognize that not all items are negotiable.

6) First, the items that are **negotiable** as part of the recruiting process (see Appendix A):

a) Specific teaching time and effort should be described. This is particularly so for those involved in medical student and/or postgraduate courses. Teaching may involve residents, fellows, master candidates, PhD candidates, or medical students, or a combination. How many hours will be involved? If the new faculty member is a PhD and is expected to establish a vibrant funded research program, will educational teaching responsibilities be deferred or moderated, and if so, for how long? Will the subseqent unanticipated lack of successful research funding and/or disappointing clinical activities, trigger the assignment of more educational responsibilities, and if so how much and what type?

b) What are the research expectations? How soon is extramural funding to be accomplished, and at what percentage of salary support? Does the expected percentage of grant salary support change with increase of academic rank and/or time at the AHC? What are the AHC's policies for senior authorship, lead authorship, and principal investigator (PI) vs. co-PI?

c) If clinical activities are part of the new faculty responsibilities, they also need to be specific. How many half- days of clinical-office patient activity are expected? If a surgical discipline, how many days per week of operating room time will be blocked-booked for this faculty member's use? As both clinical office appointment time and surgical OR needs will increase over the ramping-up months, what will be the timeline and incremental increase in resource assignment? What metrics (and for each metric, what level) will be used for measurement of clinical productivity—RVU (relative value units), dollars of billings, dollars collected, patient satisfaction scores—or a combination of these?

d) Salary levels, both start-up and once "under way," must be detailed. For guidelines on salary levels, the AAMC documents for salary levels at AHCs may be very helpful, as these data are specific for research faculty, for clinical faculty by academic rank, for geographic area, and for private and for public institutions. In the offer letter, avoid the use of the term *guarantee*, which has legal implications, committing the AHC and/or Department to an unreasonable salary level in the face of major economic changes for the AHC or because of poor productivity by the faculty member in obtaining grants or being less clinically productive. If the new faculty member wants assurance as to a stable salary, the following language is often helpful. "Your salary for the first (one, two, three) years will be at $XXX level. Thereafter you will participate in the faculty practice plan for faculty involved in (research, clinical) activity. Attached is the appropriate document for those details." Usually clinical faculty will need only one year to get the patient care activity under way with revenue, unlike the basic scientist, who will take at least three years to obtain some grant funding.

e) What other resource commitments will be provided, such as laboratory bench space (if relevant), staff support, or liability insurance coverage for clinical activity?

f) Should be specific on items such as ownership of computers, lab equipment, accounts receivable, etc.

7) There are many items for the offer letter that are **not negotiable** (see Appendix B). The author recommends that these items be a separate document attached to the offer letter, with the suggested title of "Standard Terms of Faculty Employment."

a) The language in the offer letter in the Standard Terms of Faculty Employment section should be carefully crafted by the Dean's Office and the Office of Counsel. Instructions to the Chair from the AHC should specify that these Standard Terms cannot be modified unless specifically detailed and cleared by both the Dean and the Office of Counsel. Some of the items that need to be addressed in these Standard Terms are:

b) For recruits who will have clinical responsibilities, the licensure, insurance panel responsibilities, and the timing thereof by the faculty candidate are essential to detail. These will vary from state to state, including issues of reciprocity. Do note that these licensure and similar issues in some states are very complex and difficult for graduates of medical schools and residency programs outside the United States (except Canada in some circumstances). This has been historically compounded in some clinical specialties by the inability of foreign potential clinical faculty to sit for American Board of Medical Specialties (ABMS) board-certifying examinations in the absence of an ACGME-accredited residency-training program. Recently, this latter factor might not be applicable and merits confirmation by the specific ABMS Board. It must be crystal clear to the new faculty member what his/her responsibilities are in these licensure and privilege processes, and if available, what AHC personnel he/she should contact for assistance.

c) **For clinicians, new faculty should begin the sequence of licensure, facility privileges, and insurance panel acceptance six to eight months before starting employment** if undue financial pressures are to be avoided for the AHC and the Department. The reasons are as follows. Depending on the state, licensure may take many months to achieve. All hospitals and outpatient surgical centers will require licensure before performing the due diligence for privileges, and this can take weeks or even months. Usually both licensure and facility privileges must be in place before the potential faculty member can request placement on the approved panels of third-party carriers. This sequence can easily consume six to eight months. An additional factor of which Chairs must be aware, beyond the delays imposed by licensure and by AHC institutional credentialing, is that most insurance third-party's reimbursements will lag four weeks to many months in paying for charges.

d) If ongoing clinical activity is expected, the Standard Terms offer letter document should specify the need for the licensure to be maintained in good standing, obtaining the appropriate ABMS certification and subspecialty certification (if applicable), the timeline for this credentialing, and the need to comply with all the recredentialing requirements of the applicable ABMS Board.

e) Moving expense information should include, consistent with that AHC's policy, reimbursement for personal expenses and/ or professional equipment and/or student transfers, and the required documentation for these (often best using a web link).

f) Potential new faculty should be informed about standing AHC policies and regulations. The information can be provided via website links; this is advisable, for as AHC policies and regulations are upgraded, these changes will be in the links, avoiding the need to rewrite the standard terms. Option, track, and tenure considerations are of importance and usually detailed in an AHC document dealing with faculty regulations. There is the need for compliance with AHC/University regulations and policies on intellectual property, on technology transfer, on conflict of interest, and all of the other specifications in the regulations of the faculty policies and procedures. The offer letter *must not* deviate from these AHC policies, as this will create the potential for major legal difficulties going forward.

g) Ethical behavior requirements and AHC actions that will be taken if these are violated should be referenced (usually an intranet link to AHC policies and procedures) up to and including immediate termination of all appointments, even revocation of tenure. Such ethical violations might include, but not be limited to: plagiarism, falsification of laboratory data, fraudulent publications, falsification of medical records, criminal convictions, censure by state licensing boards, loss of medical licensure, violence, harassment, or child pornography.

> *"The palest ink is better than the best memory."*
> —CHINESE PROVERB

The well written offer letter should be friendly, specific, and accurately reflect all the prior discussions among the candidate, the Chair, the Dean, and the others involved. The Standard Terms are not harsh: if a faculty candidate does not wish to abide by University and AHC policies, or does not want to agree to ethical behavior, how much better to find out in time to negate the recruitment. The portions of the offer letter crafted by the Chair, specific to this recuit and vetted by the Office of Counsel and the Dean, should simply accurately reflect all the discussions previously covered and agreed upon during the recruiting process.

Be a Leader
Make a Difference
Enjoy!

CHAPTER 27

Retaining Excellent Faculty

*"Knowing is not enough, we must apply.
Willing is not enough, we must do."*
—GOETHE

*"The least deviation from truth will be multiplied
later."*
—ARISTOTLE

Professionally and personally happy faculty are much easier to retain. In the author's experience, appreciation and acknowledgment of professional competence and accomplishment, robust mentoring and career development programs, and a happy home life are far more powerful retention factors than simple financial rewards. Proactive steps are needed to avoid the scene of "the grass is greener on other side of the fence" for excellent faculty. These proactive steps start with the initial recruitment (see chapter 26). The ease and success of retention is to a large extent predicated on:

1) Astute and effective initial recruiting of the faculty member

2) Prudent due diligence at time of initial recruit

3) Accurate, specific, detailed, and nonadversarial initial offer letter that served as:

   a) A discussion agenda of items resulting in a clear understanding between the AHC and the new faculty member of what was expected by both the AHC and the new faculty member

b) A template for the initial career in the Department, a template that both the Chair and the new faculty member can use to monitor and mentor progress

c) A clear outline of AHC resources committed and faculty performance expected

4) Excellent mentoring of the new faculty member. This should be:

a) One-on-one within the Department

b) With others across the AHC

c) By facilitating the national contacts for the new faculty member from the beginning

5) Successful facilitation of the new faculty member's interdigitation and collaboration with other faculty in the Department and across the Medical Center. The faculty member with fire in belly, energetic with enthusiasm, and a team player who has successfully established productive collaborative linkages across the Medical Center with other productive faculty is usually a "happy camper" who will be enthusiastic to remain and grow in the AHC—and hence retention is win-win.

6) The faculty member was initially added to the faculty to fill a specific Departmental and AHC need and is a net positive value to the AHC. Personal gratification with a personal sense of being respected and valued is a hugely positive motivator in professional satisfaction.

7) The faculty member recognizes the collaborative and nurturing environment. If sincere mentoring has been provided to nurture and mentor the faculty member's career, both locally and nationally, this faculty member, whom the AHC/Department wants to retain and promote, will recognize that his/her career advancement can occur smoothly and successfully at the AHC without the need to move in order to achieve future career growth.

8) The faculty member's family is happily settled in the community.

> *"Let our advance worrying become advance thinking and planning."*
> —WINSTON CHURCHILL

The preceding attributes of the recruiting process and the early career at the AHC in the Department are excellent predictors of successful win-win painless faculty retention and subsequent promotion.

A faculty member who is disillusioned and dissatisfied with the initial term will be exceedingly difficult to retain. Rarely is it justified to commit excess institutional resources to retain this individual. It is usually better to utilize those incremental resources for a new recruit or to reallocate to other productive and happy faculty.

1) In the absence of institutional involvement, in the absence of feeling appreciated, in the absence of meaningful involvement on mission-based teams, rich salary packages do not buy the long-term faculty allegiance to academic mission, commitment to excellence, or productivity.

2) There are certain warning signs that the faculty member will be difficult to retain, and perhaps not worth the resources to retain.

   a) He/she demonstrates the two almost always malignant early warning signs: 1) being overly concerned about "me"; 2) being focused unduly on personal salary issues.

   b) He/she has not been enthusiastic, and perhaps has openly resisted building the concept of "Department team."

3) If a new faculty member has exhibited these warning characteristics, it is ill-advised to spend resources to retain that faculty member,

hoping that with time he/she: a) will mature; b) will realize his/her potential; or c) will change personality.

If the Chair and the AHC have the fortunate situation of an excellent recruit followed by mentoring and an excellent early-career trajectory, retention and appropriate promotion is the prudent course to be undertaken with enthusiasm, to make it a win-win for the faculty member, the Department, and the AHC. This is also certainly true for the midcareer faculty, who usually are being considered for promotion to Professor, sometimes with tenure as well. Remember that it is often/usually more expensive to recruit an excellent new person than to invest in retaining the best and the brightest.

1) If the Department and AHC are committed to retain the faculty member, and if indeed any departure would be "a lateral move" for that faculty member, or even a promotion at another AHC, what is the prudent course of action? Waiting until the potentially departing faculty member has an attractive recruitment offer from another AHC puts the Chair in the dynamic of "playing catch-up."

2) The Chair/Center Director and AHC Senior Leadership are well-advised to be proactive in the retention plans, plans put in place well before the end of the current academic appointment.

> *"The first responsibility of a leader is to define reality. The last is to say thank you. In between, the leader is a servant."*
> —MAX DEPREE

a) Money is usually not as key as fulfillment through "job satisfaction," being appreciated, having responsibilities, and being acknowledged and praised for efforts and results (see chapters 19 and 24).

RETAINING EXCELLENT FACULTY

b) Fostering linkages with other Departments and Centers/ Programs, including an increasing role in research, clinical initiatives, and administration, will equate to "I value/ appreciate you and what you will do in the future, which with our support will be bigger and better even than all your present accomplishments."

c) Get the Dean and/or hospital CEO involved, which shows that he/she is really noticed and appreciated at the highest levels of the AHC, not just the Department; also the Chair can give significant institutional administrative/task force/work group/ think tank assignments. "This will better position you sometime in the future for a much bigger role" equates to "maybe some day you'll be my successor as Chair" (do this for only very few faculty, so pick carefully).

d) Pay raise is a consequence of the above; hence, it is a reward for accomplishments, not a bribe to try to curry favor.

e) One powerful retention tool is mentoring, not just talking about it; mentor the faculty member with roles of increasing responsibility. If the Department Chair identifies faculty with outstanding attitude, good judgment, team-player abilities, and solid talent, assign this faculty member real responsibility, with the necessary authority and the accompanying accountability. This may be in teaching, research, clinical care, and/or administration. In those endeavors, the faculty member should be mentored, either by the Chair or by another senior-faculty star.

f) Facilitate the appointment of this faculty member to important committees within the Department, across the AHC, and nationally. This will foster new-idea formation with the resultant creativity benefiting the Department and the AHC. Most important, it will increase the career satisfaction of this faculty member, who knows that he/she is making a difference.

> *"Most folks are about as happy as they make their minds up to be."*
> —Abraham Lincoln

g) Foster the faculty career by interdigitation and interrelationships with other faculty in other Departments at the AHC. This greatly expands the faculty member's horizon and contacts, usually results in increasing productivity, and sends a powerfully positive message to the faculty member. Importantly, it is also a network for that faculty member that is very hard to replicate at another AHC and thus facilitates retention.

3) In doing all of the above, in addition to enhancing faculty retention, the current Chair is accomplishing:

a) The creation of a real leadership team within the Department

b) The nurturing of "in utero" potential future internal candidate for the Chair successor

c) The development of a stronger and better-balanced Department

d) The establishment of trusted members of the Department who can lead and solve "smaller" problems within the Department, freeing the Chair's time to deal with the "real big" issues

e) This assignment of opportunity and responsibility by the Chair to the more junior or midcareer faculty is not limited to positions within the Department, or even AHC-wide multiple Department committees or task forces. This can be extended nationally. For example:

i) The Chair is asked to join a committee in a national organization. Rather than become overcommitted, the Chair can, and should, respond, "This committee and effort is important. I will be hard-pressed to give it the time it deserves, and I have an outstanding faculty member in my

Department who would be perfect for that. The name is XXX; let me tell you about XXX and why he/she would be a perfect fit. His/her e-mail address is…"

    ii) A similar and analogous strategy also is effective with requests that come to the Chair for coauthorship or editorial responsibilities. The Chair should suggest the appropriate bright member of the Department for this authorship. This is another way to mentor, through nurturing, moving the early- and midcareer faculty forward on the national scene.

4) The above strategy will make it very clear to these junior and mid-career faculty that their career can advance locally and nationally without the need to move to another AHC.

In spite of the above, some outstanding faculty will be targeted for major leadership in other AHCs (i.e., they are "Chair material," and unless the current Chair is stepping aside or leaving, they "have no choice" in their career other than to leave). In this situation, the Chair should:

1) Be gracious. To do so:

    a) May set the stage for the person to return at some future point as the successor to the Chair or to another senior position

    b) Creates a strong ally on the national scene from another AHC

    c) Will enhance the departing person's opinion of the AHC, the Department and the Chair

2) Retain the grants and accounts receivable if possible for the Department/Center. There are multiple factors here to consider, often influenced by University or AHC policies and by federal regulations. For example, it may be possible to retain grants, especially with multiple investigators, but less so for single-investigator awards. In contrast to the single-grant awardee, for awards such as center grants, program project grants, and awards granted to large teams of faculty at the AHC, it is more often that

these grants must be retained because the AHC and the Department need to protect the other faculty at the institution. There are other resources that the Chair may wish to retain in the Department, such as: a) unique research resources generated by the departing investigator; b) transgenic mice and cell lines; and c) intellectual property. Note that interinstitutional agreements will need to be generated if the investigator wishes to use the intellectual property at the new AHC. Another factor to consider for departing research faculty is the ownership of equipment. Equipment bought on active NIH grants may be moved, but all other equipment usually remains. Note that it is feasible to permit departing faculty to "buy" current equipment at a fair market price (depreciated as appropriate for age, value, and cost); this purchasing arrangement is usually accomplished by the departing faculty using start-up funds from the new AHC employer.

3) Try to structure the departure details so he/she can help identify and work with an internal successor to enhance a smooth transition. If there is no strong internal person, the departing faculty member may well know of excellent external candidates to be contacted as part of a search process. If all is done gracefully, the departing faculty member will be very valuable in not only identifying, but also in recruiting someone he/she knows who might be a great addition to the Department and a successor to the vacated position.

4) Have a social event to thank and acknowledge prior contributions of the person leaving. Do this appropriately modestly, in order that other faculty don't think, "Gee, the only way to really get noticed and thanked is to leave."

Be a Leader
Make a Difference
Enjoy!

CHAPTER 28

Faculty with Inappropriate Performance or Behavior

"People are the most difficult thing in the world to change."

—GENA SHOWALTER

"Everyone has a photographic memory. Some just don't have film."

—STEPHEN WRIGHT

Just as the Chair is responsible for recruiting the best and the brightest faculty, and for retaining those faculty who have proved to be the best and the brightest, the Chair is also responsible to prune the faculty who are not performing to expectations, are exhibiting inappropriate or disruptive behavior, or have ethical or compliance issues. This is one of the most difficult and challenging tasks for an effective Chair.

There are many possible scenarios requiring this Chair action. There are several categories of faculty who "have" to leave or should leave. In some situations there is time for a measured due-diligence process; these are usually poor performance over time. In other situations, action needs to be immediate; these occur with matters of criminal behavior such as murder, child incest, rape, etc.

1)   Faculty for whom retirement is prudent, include those faculty who are progressively less productive. Of interest is that the more astute

and gracious the faculty member, the more the team player, the more apt he/she is to step forward and volunteer to assume another role needed by the Department, or to commensurately decrease his/her salary, or even to retire. The troubles arise with those faculty who lack self insight or faculty who full well recognize the problems but look upon their faculty appointment and salary as a "right," a "financial safety net," and almost as "an institutional Social Security Program." This latter situation is especially difficult if the faculty member: a) is tenured; b) has prior letters/documents referencing a "guaranteed salary"; and/or c) has a disability with potential application of the American with Disability Act.

"Potential has a shelf life."
—MARGARET ATWOOD

2) Junior or midcareer faculty (ranks of Assistant Professors and Associate Professors), with time-limited appointments at that specific rank for a specific number of years, whom the Chair and ELT do not believe merit ongoing faculty status should be neither reappointed at end of current appointment nor should they be promoted if there is an impending "up or out" decision. The Chair cannot make arbitrary, sudden decisions, but must gather facts, go through the steps outlined in this chapter, and document, document, document. There are many reasons or situations resulting in the need to either not reappoint or to not promote. It usually involves some combination of lack of productivity and/or poor attitudes in teaching, research, and/or clinical care. Terminations in midappointment are much more difficult, involving potentially substantive legal issues; for these, the Office of Counsel and the Dean need to be involved from the beginning.

> *"Man is a creature made at the end of the week when God was tired."*
> —Mark Twain

3) Reasons other than lack of productivity for faculty to merit neither reappointment nor promotion are several and include:

a) The faculty member's research may no longer align with the research focus and strategies of the Department, or the research substance may be of insufficient quality for realistic expectations for ongoing extramural funding.

b) The faculty member's clinical activity and expertise is in an area no longer part of the vision and mission of the Department and the AHC.

4) Situations that are behavioral and/or ethical are complex from both legal and human resource perspectives. These problems may even generate issues of faculty, resident, staff, or patient safety. Some of these behaviors may be so egregious as to merit termination in midappointment; others may be less overt, just under that threshold. Examples of these nonacademic issues include but are not limited to:

a) Faculty who are abusive verbally to faculty, staff, residents, and other Departmental personnel. This may take several forms—unwarranted belittling and humiliating comments to individuals in front of others, shouting at others, and invading others' personal space

b) Faculty member who spreads false gossip (can border on actual slander) about one faculty member behind that person's back with the purpose of tearing someone else down, often to advance the gossiper's position

c) Faculty who are inappropriate and very poor role models for residents, fellows, and students. These actions tend to fall into two categories—very poor judgment (taking residents to strip joints or gambling sites) or issues of ethics (see below).

d) Faculty exhibiting poor ethics and compliance issues are not common, but distressingly this does happen. Examples include falsification of laboratory data, falsification in operative notes, altering patient consent forms (after the surgery, or after the consent for human subjects research), or inappropriate billing for clinical services such as unbundling or upcoding. Very distressing are faculty who perform complex clinical procedures when simpler ones would be just as beneficial or even better for the patient, or even more egregious, faculty who operate when it is not necessary.

e) There are some faculty with "charm and good personality" who may be popular but not productive. These include individuals who have no grants and are making little or poor efforts to get grant funding, and/or are ineffective teachers and/or have little or no clinical productivity whether measured by RVU or by revenues. In summary, these pleasant individuals have lost value to the institution and "schmooze and coast." These situations can occur regardless of the faculty age or duration on faculty.

f) Faculty who, although busy in clinical activity, have not maintained the level of clinical competence expected. There may be patterns of errors in diagnosis or surgical complications.

> *"An appeaser is one who feeds a crocodile—hoping it will eat him last."*
> —WINSTON CHURCHILL

The Chair needs to keep a Department file on each faculty member. Hopefully these are replete with excellent reports. However, such will not be the case for the faculty being considered in this chapter. For the troublesome faculty, the Chair must follow process, must document,

document, document, and is well-advised to keep both the Dean and the Office of Counsel informed. There are several component steps, each important, and each can be time-consuming.

This up-front procedural time is well invested and will usually be much less than the time required later for the Chair to correct the mistakes of omission; in fact, these omissions may not be retrospectively correctable, in which situation the Chair's hands may be tied, thus precluding proper steps by the AHC to separate these "bad actor" faculty. These steps for the Chair include, but are not limited to, the Chair being careful to:

1) Be aware of the performance of each faculty member (or in large Departments, each Division chief, who in turn must be aware of all the faculty performance in his/her Division).

2) Meet with all faculty, but take extra time and care with the faculty member of concern because of performance and other worrisome issues to discuss (see chapter 24 regarding these conversations):

   a) What was and is expected of faculty members and where/how this faculty member is not meeting expectations and how and where the person is deficient

   b) What remediation is expected, how, and over what time frame

   c) Who will provide mentoring of the delinquent faculty member; how and by what metrics the progress will be monitored and measured

   d) The timeline for improvement, and how will the improvement or lack thereof be measured—as an "all or nothing" matter (one more such occurrence and the faculty member is released); or is the improvement expected in increments over time (e.g., improvement in clinical RVUs, obtaining of extramural research funding, better teaching reviews). **The Chair should remember that it is easier to manage that which can be measured.**

   e) Schedule of follow-up meetings for the Chair with the faculty member

f) These meetings should be in the presence of another person appropriate to the situation (maybe a program administrator, or a senior faculty member, especially if it is the person who will mentor and monitor the faculty member being remediated)

g) Note that meticulous and ongoing documentation is essential: all the meetings with the Chair must be followed with a memo to the faculty member, with a copy to the faculty file, detailing the substance of the meeting. Often it is prudent, even essential, that these memos be vetted by the Office of Counsel; in fact, the author would often meet with the Office of Counsel, discuss the meeting to be held with the faculty member, and have a draft of the memo in mind to serve as a guideline for the meeting. After each meeting, two copies of the memo should be made, one for the faculty member to retain, and one for the faculty member to cosign in agreement as to the substance of the meeting; this is the copy of the memo, which is then placed in the Department's faculty file. All meetings with the mentor/monitors must be similarly documented.

3) Hold sequential serial meetings, tailored to the progress or lack thereof.

4) The Chair should involve key individuals outside the Department:

a) The Dean, to keep him/her apprised and up to date so that he/she will not get blindsided later on—and importantly to get advice as matters evolve

b) The Office of Counsel, to review all notes to file and advise on wording of all memos to the faculty member

> "Ears that do not listen to advice, accompany the head when it is chopped off."
> —AFRICAN PROVERB

5) There are several situations of faculty termination:

a) One solution occurs if and when the faculty member is lost to recruitment to another AHC. These faculty are usually productive, with enough national profile to be a recruiting target. The recruiting AHC either is unaware of the behavioral (EQ) issues, or believes "it is just the poor current environment, and we know how to do it better."

b) Another favorable solution is if the difficult faculty member is the spouse of a good faculty member in the same or another Department who is recruited away.

c) If the faculty member is due for reappointment or up-or-out promotion, the Chair can use the AHC's policies and regulations for the faculty (or the promotion processes and requirements) to let the "system" decide objectively on academic issues that this faculty member does not qualify for promotion and therefore must leave the AHC as an "up or out." This up-or-out solution will work for academically nonproducers, but usually not for EQ issues.

There are faculty who will fail all attempts at remediation. Sometimes the ongoing shortcomings are so damaging or flagrant that this faculty member needs to be "fired" midappointment for cause. This is very important to accomplish, must be carefully done, and is a field full of land mines. In that situation, from the beginning it is mandatory for the Chair to involve the Dean and the Office of Counsel. There are so many variations of this situation that "when you've seen one, you've seen one." In an attempt to cluster these, the following may be helpful.

1) The Chair saw this problem coming, and has been proactive, involving all the steps and the actions listed earlier in this chapter:

a) Repeated meetings with the faculty member, with another person present, at which time the Chair reviewed problem(s), laid out corrections required, provided proper counseling by the Chair or by someone else qualified to do so, and was clear about consequences for failing to improve (including decrease in responsibilities, decrease in salary, and "firing" before the end of the current appointment)

b) Paper trail documentation of each meeting with details of each of the above points, and a letter to the faculty member either a) outlining points or b) a copy of the Chair's notes to the faculty file. Use the Office of Counsel for wording assistance of these letters and notes to file.

c) Dean and/or hospital CEO has been informed so they are not blindsided

> *"I learned long ago, never to wrestle with a pig. You get dirty, and besides, the pig likes it."*
> —GEORGE BERNARD SHAW

2) Unfortunately, there are also situations where the Chair does not have the luxury of the option for measured, stepwise processes as outlined above. The faculty is found to be involved in illegal, unethical, or destructive behavior, which is such that it precludes the possibility of remedial and corrective action to permit faculty retention.

a) Examples include, but are not limited to, the situation when the Chair and AHC suddenly encounter situations of:

i) Documented sexual harassment and discrimination

ii) Faculty who accept full-time appointments with salary and benefits at more than one AHC

iii) Faculty with criminal activity such as child pornography, manslaughter, or workplace violence

b) Unfortunately, any of these situations can surface suddenly, without warning, and hence, there may be little or no prior documentation. It is essential to move quickly and involve the Dean, the CEO, and the Office of Counsel.

c) The details of actions required are complex legally, and the Chair will need to follow and comply with the cold legal facts. Because of the variations in AHC policies and regulations with dictated due-process procedures (especially if issues of tenure are present), compounded by variations in state laws, the charged faculty member may need academic appointments and privileges "suspended" until the termination is effective. During this suspension, is the faculty member to be paid? This is a matter to be decided consistent with AHC policy and with essential input by the Dean and the Office of Counsel. Issues of "with or without salary and benefits" are complex, and it is necessary for the Chair to pursue strategies and documentations with the Office of Counsel to successfully navigate University and AHC policies, and comply with all federal and state laws.

d) Although it is counterintuitive in the "court of common sense," in some situations, limited-term appointments of two to five years are considered "tenured" for those few years, and hence, although hospital privileges can be immediately suspended for clinicians, removal/dismissal of academic appointment/employment may be controversial unless the offer letter and prior reappointment letters contain key phrases referring to this type of scenario and the consequences for such behavior (see chapter 26, Appendix A, and Appendix B for details).

3) For all the behaviors and situations above, the resolution is much more complex if the faculty member has an academic appointment with unlimited tenure. This can be very difficult. There will be many issues for the Chair to navigate with AHC CEO, the Dean, and in-house counsel.

a) For the specific AHC, what are the due-diligence appeals processes available to a faculty member whose unlimited tenure is proposed for withdrawal?

b) How long does this appeals process take?

c) Does the AHC have to provide salary and benefits during this process, and if so, at prior levels or at reduced levels? These financial obligations may be especially difficult, as often the event(s) precipitating the proposed "firing and termination of tenure" comes from egregious faculty behavior that precludes that faculty member from any clinical or research activity that might generate income during the appeal processes within the AHC.

> *"Support bacteria. They're the only culture some people have."*
> —STEVEN WRIGHT

4) What should the research, clinical, teaching, and/or educational responsibilities of the faculty member be during these possible processes of termination, whether it is from decision not to reappoint, a decision to terminate midterm a time-limited appointment, or termination of unlimited tenure?

a) For clinical activity, are there quality and patient safety issues?

b) If research activity, is integrity of data an issue?

c) If research studies with human subjects are involved, is subject or patient safety an issue?

d) If the research involves the use of animals, is animal safety an issue?

e) How and when must external funding sources be notified?

f) In educational activity, is student safety an issue? In situations with assault, sexual harassment, or diversity issues involving students, residents, and/or fellows, obviously these faculty contacts cannot be permitted. What about situations harder to define clearly, such as poor role- modeling?

5) Just as the precise and inclusive nature of the proper offer letter (see chapter 26, Appendix A, Appendix B) helps ensure excellent early faculty performance and then makes much easier the successful retention and/or promotion efforts, so too that initial offer letter and the annual performance review documents greatly facilitate the smooth departure of underperforming or unethical faculty. These letters and documents in their specificity and inclusiveness pinpoint the problems. The faculty member has fallen short of expectations. Examples of key wordings for those expectations are usually included in the Standard Terms component of the prudent offer letter and/ or the portions of the offer letter (or the reappointment or promotion letter) as crafted by the Chair (see chapter 26):

a) "You are expected to perform XYZ RVU units."

b) "You are required to maintain proper and current licensure credentials."

c) "By the third year of this appointment, you are to have xxx% of your salary covered by extramural grant-funding sources."

d) "This appointment is contingent upon ethical behavior, compliance with all regulations of the AHC, and the absence of any activity resulting in criminal or felony convictions."

e) The offer letter and subsequent letters to the faculty avoid all references to the salary-term "guarantee." Phrasing possibilities avoiding that term include:

i) "Your salary for the next #Z years will be $XXX per year, paid in monthly installments. You will be eligible for productivity bonuses, in accordance with the policies and metrics as detailed in the faculty compensation plan."

ii) For faculty who have been granted tenure, wording is very helpful, such as: "Your salary will have a tenure-base component of $XXX per year, paid in monthly installments. Your total annual salary will be $YYY per year, paid in monthly installments. In addition, you will be eligible for productivity bonuses, in accordance with the policies and metrics as detailed in the faculty compensation plan. As you know and as has been previously documented for you in writing, tenure is granted based upon prior academic productivity and with the understanding that the faculty member will continue with commensurate academic productivity. Should that not be the case, salary levels may increase or decrease, and may decrease below the tenure base; in this unlikely possibility, appeals and grievance procedures are available as outlined in the faculty compensation plan."

6) The letter to the faculty member advising him/her of separation from the AHC must be crafted by the Office of Counsel with the Chair, approved by the Dean, and be based upon the details in the Chair's and Department's faculty file. The more closely all of the items in this chapter have been followed, the better the termination letter and the smoother the separation.

One specific situation not included in this chapter is that of the spouse or partner who is leaving the Department to follow his/her significant other to another AHC. This individual may be a valuable or marginal faculty member, but the Chair is not initiating the departure.

Be a Leader
Make a Difference
Enjoy!

CHAPTER 29

The Balancing Tightrope of Conflicting Visions and Strategies of the AHC and the Department

> *"It is the mark of an educated mind to be able to entertain a thought without accepting it."*
> —ARISTOTLE

> *"Efforts and courage are not enough without purpose and direction."*
> —JOHN F. KENNEDY

The academic Chair should have an important role in collaboration with the Senior Leadership in the planning of the strategic goals of the AHC. At times these strategic goals may mesh with and complement those of his/her Department. At other times these AHC strategies may not fall in line with what the Chair believes to be important goals for his/her Department. Examples of these conflicts are what clinical service lines are to be emphasized or which research priorities will receive AHC hard-money support.

Unfortunately and distressingly common, the Chair will find him/herself in the difficult position when what he/she knows is best for the Department runs counter to the proposed actions of Senior Leadership for the overall AHC. This may be a fundamental difference in vision and mission or may involve requests to deliver more with fewer resources.

One example of this latter situation would be demands from the AHC for more medical student teaching without incremental salary support for those faculty and at the same time demanding more clinical output and/or more grant funding. Another example is the reduction of salary and benefit budgets for the clinical activities of faculty at the very time these same faculty are supposed to increase clinical activity. This may well have a very adverse impact on clinical faculty retention at the very time when these faculty are necessary both to maintain the overall clinical mission and to sustain hospital survival.

The economic climate is not a constant to be taken for granted. At the time this is being written, the challenges facing the health-care system and the AHC are perhaps more harsh than at any time in the history of what might be called modern medicine. Leaving aside political parties and honest differences in possible solutions, the pressures are multiple, and include, but are not limited to, those detailed in the following list for clinical care, education, and research.

With limited resources, in each situation the Chair faces a "conflicted balancing act" with other Chairs competing for limited AHC resources. Senior Leadership will be determined to deliver the best overall result possible, yet recognize that many good and/or excellent deliverables may not be possible. This is very difficult for the Chair if one of his/her programs is a casualty. Data from Departmental successes to the present time may be powerfully persuasive; success breeds success (see Appendix D).

The ability of AHC to treat so many conditions as a tertiary and quaternary referral center for clinical care, the broad scope of exciting but very costly basic research, and the costs of education exceed available resources, resources that must be wisely used. Some examples of these pressures and challenges are:

1) **Pressures of clinical care challenges:**

    a) Many more individuals needing care

b) An aging population with many more senior citizens, whose heath-care needs and end-of-life care needs can be and usually are very expensive

c) The ability of patient care providers with all the new advances to treat many conditions previously not treatable, and even to prolong meaningful life. But all of these faculty clinical efforts will increase the costs for interventional care and at the same time, by prolonging life, will increase the size of the elderly pool.

d) The emergence of "clinical quality metrics" and "performance metrics," which are to be linked to hospital and physician reimbursements. Unfortunately, although these will most certainly be used by third-party payors, predictably these may not correlate with the expertise of quality care. Patient-satisfaction survey results often relate to matters of recognized importance such as waiting times, ambiance of facilities, etc., but unfortunately may *not* correlate with critical issues such as the quality of care, the expertise of the clinical team, and the long-term morbidity and mortality data.

e) Defining and then implementing the distinctions between what *can* be done to treat and help the patient vs. what *should* be done for treatment in all age groups; and, very importantly, by whom are those decisions to be made—the government at state level, the government at federal level, the insurance industry, a local health-care "system," or the working together of the individual physician/patient/patient's family?

f) How in this environment with these imposed external forces is the individual physician to achieve the goal of delivering ethical care to the individual patient, consistent with the time-honored Hippocratic Oath?

g) Is the most effective and efficient health care model:

i) Many more primary care physicians, fewer specialists?

ii) More nurse practitioners and physician assistants making the primary care physician more productive with more patients cared for by fewer primary care physicians, and increasing the number of specialists to deliver targeted definitive care?

h) How, and is it even possible, to link the patient (consumer) with the payor for health care? At present, the payors for health care are any combination of the federal government, the state governments, and industry (via health care insurance benefits). With these large, impersonal economic entities taking the role of the "consumer," how can the interests, values, and desires of the individual patient and patient cohorts be protected?

i) Added to these problems is the increasing number of underinsured patients (from large unexpected co-pay responsibilities) and/or limitations in physician and hospital panels secondary to the implementation of the Affordable Care Act (ACA). With the ACA in place, hospitals and AHCs will more and more become the safety net, but very possibly with reduced and inadequate reimbursements to the AHC "system" of physicians, clinics, emergency rooms, and inpatient census.

j) In response to these pressures, the answer to lower health-care costs is *not* simply "population health with better preventative care," because the death rate is still eventually 1:1. The terminal illness may be delayed, but it will occur and with the associated costs. Ideally, all people would live healthy, long lives with low cost, and then suddenly die at low cost. That is not reality unless society considers assisted suicide, and/or rationing care for the elderly, and/or earlier augmented palliative to hospice care. One of the most successful health-care initiatives over the past two centuries has been the vaccination and immunization programs. These have prevented untold suffering and prolonged greatly population life spans. They may not save money, however. As Willard Gaylin (12) once said, "Those who would have died from polio or measles or pertussis will grow up to be a very expensive old men or women." To paraphrase, every younger person who does not die suddenly from infection lives to become a very expensive old person. Obviously vaccination programs are very essential and should be mandatory unless excepted for a specific medical reason. These programs will save costs and decrease suffering now, are laudatory, and should be sustained—but will these programs result in higher costs in the distant future with more people surviving to be elderly?

k) All of these items above put enormous pressure with resultant conflicts on the AHC Senior Leadership and the Departmental Chairs on how best to allocate limited resources for patient care—young vs. old, population medicine vs. the individual patient, expensive new innovations vs. older, less expensive (and perhaps less effective) treatments.

l) These conflicts extend within the AHC—resources for cardiac care vs. resources for dementia care, resources for trauma care vs. cancer, etc.

2) **Pressures from educational challenges:**

a) AHCs have been charged to educate more physicians in anticipation of a physician shortage from the increasing health-care needs of the aging population, but what and where are the resources to do this? Medical students are saddled with debts. In spite of high tuitions, AHCs recognize that the costs of medical student education exceed the tuition revenues even as faculty donate teaching-time hours. Residency programs' salary and benefits are an emerging problem with a disconnect from reality. Medical schools have been charged to educate more MDs. How shortsighted it is that funding for residency-training positions is frozen at levels from several years ago. How can it be that society, via government, says, "Educate more MDs, but we won't fund the necessary subsequent number of needed residency-training positions?" In the past and at present, these training programs have been financed primarily by federal and state government insurance reimbursements for hospitals, but: a) this funding is being constricted; b) the federal government has not increased the number of residency slots to be funded in many years; c) medical schools are responding to the need to graduate more physicians to care for the increasing aging population; and d) this decrease in residency funding is occurring at the very time that more medical school graduates will be seeking residency positions.

b) Resident work-hour restrictions mandated by law may result in less resident fatigue but have not demonstrated any improvement in patient care and safety. These hour restrictions have resulted in increasing AHC costs to hire physician assistants and nurse practitioners, and may well be having a significant adverse impact on resident education in procedural specialties such as Surgery and Orthopaedics.

c) More and more, student and resident education involves simulation experiential learning with effective but very expensive computer models.

d) Thus, it is easy to see the conflicts of one Chair vs. another within the AHC as debates occur with Senior Leadership on how best to proceed. Which residencies will be retained? Which residencies will be increased in number of positions, and which will have fewer slots? As an AHC's Senior Leadership debate which educational programs to support for resident education, Chairs of less-favored disciplines are conflicted. For example, by what measure can it be said that training for physicians in suicide prevention is more or less important than training for physicians in the care of mothers and infants in premature deliveries?

e) There is a strong pressure to reduce the cost of education. This includes a move toward online learning. Will this hinder or enhance the expensive but necessary one-on-one teaching with role-modeling of the doctor-patient interface by the experienced clinician mentor? Will the use of more online learning make it more complex to create new revenue-generating course offerings such as new MS degree programs and certificate programs?

3) **Pressures from research challenges:**

a) Many research programs that have been traditionally well-funded are challenged to obtain ever more competitive continuing funding from government sources, be it NIH, NCI, and/or the Department of Defense.

b) AHCs are educating PhDs who are gifted in research, at the very time that funding for research is decreasing and therefore, the junior-level academic appointments are fewer and more competitive. The average researcher's age at the time of receiving the first NIH R01 has increased to over forty.

c) Industrial sources for research financial support is one potential funding opportunity, but there are issues associated with this. Many pharmaceutical and device companies are eliminating or markedly decreasing internal research and development divisions and are resorting to outsourcing. This outsourcing may be to research components of an AHC, and if so, the research-intense AHCs are all competing for these same dollars. There are mixed messages from the federal government on these industry-AHC alliances. On the one hand some federal agencies are promoting "public-private partnerships." But at the same time some federal agencies are becoming rather aggressive in demanding detailed financial reporting by the investigators and by their AHCs in matters that might involve financial conflict of interest. This government pressure to challenge and oversee the management of possible conflict of interest may well result in a restraint to industry-supported AHC research—both from the contraction of industry itself, and from a reduction in the interest of industry to invest in the outsourcing of research and development. Other challenges to these industry-AHC relationships are the negotiating of intellectual property issues (see chapter 30) and the policies related to publication freedoms.

d) If the partnership between the AHC and industry is necessary and beneficial, how is it best to develop management plans for the potential conflicts of interest (see chapter 32)?

In summary of the challenges, within the context of all these challenges, how is it best for the AHC to respond? AHCs are being asked to do more with less:

1) Educate more physicians, but with inadequate funding sources
2) Increase the number of resident trainees to accommodate the increasing number of new MDs but with fewer resources to do this
3) Deliver more patient care of greater complexity with fewer resources
4) Sustain cutting-edge research in the face of decreasing resources
5) Train brilliant researcher PhDs/MDPhDs without the support funding and with fewer junior faculty positions available
6) Seek other sources for educational and research funding when the traditional sources of government, of clinical hospital revenues, and of faculty practice income are all decreasing. One source is relationships between AHC and industry, but government regulations are making this difficult.

The Chair is caught in the middle. He/she knows of these challenges listed above and the associated costs with economic realities. The Chair on the positive side is also aware of opportunities and needs in his/her area that may have major positive possibilities for revenue enhancement and/ or cost management for the AHC. These visionary programs may have major near- or long-term beneficial impact for better patient care, more competitive research funding and discoveries, and intellectual property and patent possibilities. But even with these great ideas, the Chair may not be able to move forward unless these ideas are consistent with the visions of the Senior Leadership for the entire AHC. Only the Chair will know the needs, the challenges, and the opportunities locally, regionally, and/or nationally within that component of the AHC for which he/she is responsible. The Chair's ideas may deal with population and individual-patient clinical-care demands, educational needs of emerging MDs and residency trainees, and imaginative research horizons. The Chair is obligated to make the cogent, concise, and convincing presentation to the Senior Leadership and the other Chairs. The Chair cannot alone advance his/her Department, as Senior Leadership with their financial policies and control are responsible for the macroeconomics of the entire AHC, and hence have the burden of allocation and rationing of limited resources.

> *"I said, 'Somebody should do something about that.' Then I realized I am somebody."*
> —LILLY TOMLIN

Considering all of these challenges within this labyrinth, the Chair is balancing on the "tightrope of conflicts:"

1) The vision and mission of the AHC may marginalize his/her Department's needs and goals.

2) The challenge is for the Chair to espouse the role and relevance of his/her Department within the AHC, and that his/her visionary suggestions may benefit the AHC as well as the Department. This is especially win-win if several Departments with Chair collaborations come together to create imaginative, new, beneficial, and cost-effective programs that benefit the AHC and the Departments involved.

3) The opportunities and societal-population needs may exist for a Department to service a mission, but if the Department's needs and goals are not aligned with and supported by the AHC's Senior Leadership, the AHC will not provide support, and continued pursuit by the Chair will drain Departmental resources.

4) Within this situational conflict, if at all possible, the Chair needs to convince the Senior Leadership to recognize, acknowledge, and then support the Chair's vision for opportunities as a win-win for the AHC and the Department.

5) As "no money, no mission" is a hard truism, the Chair should best frame his/her proposal within the context of the idealistic merit of meeting societal needs married to the potential to deliver incremental revenue and/or to manage resources more efficiently with decreasing expenses, thus maximizing net revenues.

6) Even with these Chair efforts, Senior Leadership may decide that what might be best for the Department may not benefit the overall AHC mission.

> *"It is wise to direct your anger toward problems—*
> *not people;*
> *to focus your energies on answers—not excuses."*
> —WILLIAM ARTHUR WARD

Thus, the Department Chair/Center Director is thrust into an incredibly difficult situation, requiring the wisdom to know the best course of action to coordinate and blend the missions of the AHC and the Department and the faculty. This means the Chair needs the skill sets to gracefully and forcefully navigate the leadership path to the outcome that benefits as many stakeholders as possible. This is a situation requiring consensus building, aligning of incentives, and developing shared visions among many Departments and components of the AHC. The key is a calm, measured approach based upon integrity, fairness, facts, and persistence (see chapters 14, 15, 16, 17, 18, 19, 20, 21, 22, 23, 24, and 25).

A Chair who does not understand the preceding situation and is a self-centered Chair will not long be tolerated and will not succeed long-term, even if having initial progress. Self-interest with a focus only in his/her ideas is limiting and precludes seeing the overall AHC situation. This type of Chair is a disaster for the AHC with the philosophy of "What's mine is mine, and what's yours is mine, and you give it to me or I'll take it." Such Chairs must not be allowed to hold the AHC hostage, and are best replaced—the sooner the better in order to minimize collateral damage.

> *"Never allow a person to tell you no who doesn't have the power to say yes."*
> —ELEANOR ROOSEVELT

The balancing needed by the Chair is not limited to AHC vs. Departmental issues, but within the Department when it involves striking a balance among the missions and responsibilities of the departmental Divisions.

1) Research vs. education vs. clinical efforts all pose legitimate conflict. Time is money and resources. Time spent educating students and residents and mentoring PhD students is time not spent in clinical productivity or in conducting research or writing successful grants.

2) Most large Departments have several Divisions with areas of subexpertise. Some are financially lucrative. Some are cost centers. The academic value and patient-care importance may not parallel the cash flow. The Chair has to adjudicate these very difficult issues.

3) Across all AHCs there is a real need to develop the physician scientist. These are the uncommon and unusually talented faculty who are capable of and are recipients of major extramural

research funding, and yet at the same time are talented and astute clinicians (most often with a subspecialty area of focus). These are the gifted faculty in this era of translational research who are in such demand, and from whom the truly valuable advances in patient care will emanate. As these faculty spend significant time in research, their clinical income is compromised, especially as the subspecialty clinical focus is often underreimbursed. This leads to the real challenge for the Chair to protect the income of these valuable faculty by mobilizing resources for this purpose—but from where?

4) Within the Department, the Chair will need to create and adjudicate compensation systems. It takes the wisdom of Solomon to marry productivity incentives with shared resources.

5) The Chair needs to discern the status of the AHC's "economic pie." Is this AHC's "economic pie" growing, staying the same, or decreasing? Most likely for the foreseeable future the pie will be decreasing in total dollars at the same time as the obligations are increasing.

6) The Chair is in the middle in the allocation of resources among education, research, clinical care, community outreach, and administrative obligations. Senior Leadership may have no choice but to decrease resources, yet the Departmental faculty will plead for more resources. At the same time, other Chairs may be pleading with Senior Leadership for a shift of resources from one Department or area to another, a real challenge in the environment of a smaller pie.

Be a Leader
Make a Difference
Enjoy!

D. Other Important Issues

CHAPTER 30

The Nontraditional Roles of the Chair in Raising Revenues

"His leadership is such that he doesn't get people to follow him; he gets people to join him."
—NFL ALL-PRO STEVE TASKER, DESCRIBING COACH MARV LEVY

As is apparent to all, financial stability is one of the major challenges faced by Chairs. No longer in AHCs will transfer of clinical revenues from hospitals and/or faculty practice plans sustain the multiple missions of education, research, patient care, and community outreach. There are many other potential revenue sources, but honest creativity is required in mobilizing resources from endowment income, intellectual property and patents, technology transfer, start-up companies, and relationships with industry.

In times of financial challenges created by forces that cannot be controlled by the Chair—such as the decreasing clinical income from third-party payors, constriction of hospital budgets, and decreases in traditional research funding from the NIH, DoD, etc.—the Chair must be innovative for supplemental resources of revenue. There are several opportunities that may arise. Those will vary from Department to Department—for example, philanthropy from grateful patients may be more common in clinical Departments, while research activity is more apt to provide intellectual property possibilities.

In this area of raising revenues from nontraditional sources, the Chair usually has limited personal knowledge of what must be known and done. Hence, it is very wise for the Chair to seek and follow expert advice. Most

AHCs have developed robust offices with the necessary expertise (Office of Counsel, Office of Technology Transfer and Patents and Intellectual Property, Office of Research Administration, and Offices for Development or Advancement), and sometimes even these AHC experts may see the need to retain additional experts from outside the AHC.

There is one common fatal risk to Chairs in seeking help from these revenue sources—the naive Chair who does not recognize the need for specialized help. One such very complex area is that of intellectual property, technology transfer, and patents. The Chair will need legal and financial consultants (usually including in-depth knowledge of tax law) in any interactions with potential philanthropic donors. No matter how much a donor wants to gift to a medical cause, the tax implications and possibilities are paramount. Potential relationships with industry carry major obligations in defining and protecting intellectual property and patents—and solid advice is needed from people with expertise in the management of conflicts of interest.

> *"The greater danger for most of us lies not in setting our aim too high and falling short, but in setting our aim too low and achieving our mark."*
> —MICHELANGELO

These sources of additional revenue are considered here in more detail.

1) **Philanthropy** presents real opportunity for the missions of the AHC to benefit from the deeply positive and emotional experiences of potential donors. Some concepts are worth considering in order to maximize results:

   a) The donor will want to select the target for his/her gifting. If the donor is interested in "A," do not push the donor into "B." To do so may result in a small gift to "B," rather than a large gift to "A."

269

b) The donor may have had personal or family disease(s), treatment(s), and/or surgeries that had a profound impact. This can be a powerful donor motivator. The donor may be saying "thank you," or may want to fund programs to better understand and treat a condition that devastated him/her, personally or in the family, or close friend.

c) The donor may approach the Chair directly. Or the donor may turn to the faculty member with whom he/she interacted and/ or has been treated. This faculty member should express great appreciation and should offer to facilitate a meeting with the Chair. Neither the Chair nor the faculty member should ask for the gift or the amount. This is for the experts.

d) The Chair should sincerely thank the potential donor. Suggested wording might include, "Your interest is wonderful. The Department, Dr. XXX, and I are so very grateful that you'd like to help (find a cure for YY, learn how to best treat ZZZ). Gifting is so important, and we want to be certain to use your proposed gift just as you wish. This area of gifting is complex and with many ways to gift, each with various tax benefits. I recommend you meet with my friend here from Advancement, and perhaps you will want to involve some of your financial planners. We really want this to work for you just as you want. As part of our thank-you, we want to be certain your gift has the best possible tax benefits for you as well."

e) The Chair and the faculty member should ASAP meet with the in-house professional fundraisers, be the nomenclature "Donor Development, Development, Advancement," or some similar title. A menu of opportunities for the donor must be quickly created. Do not assume the size of the donor's intention. This list of opportunities should range from books for the library to major endowments of Chairs, Departments, special programs, etc.

f) The key roles of the Chair throughout these processes are to develop the menu of gifting opportunities and to facilitate the meetings for the potential donor(s) with all the appropriate individuals at the AHC (usually including the contact faculty member).

g) The script for the Chair should include:

  i) Thank the donor(s) for their interest.

  ii) Learn more about the positive aspects of what the donor experienced and reaffirm the sentiments.

  iii) Share information with the potential donor about the Departmental activities in that area or those areas that the donor has indicated to be of interest.

  iv) Explain how important those activities are.

  v) Throughout these meetings the Chair should reaffirm, "Your interest is fabulous, and possible donation/gifting so appreciated. We want to make certain this works out just the way you wish and is of maximum benefit to your financial planning, taxes, etc. This is so complex and with many ways to gift, each with various tax benefits."

h) Let the professional advancement people take the lead. They are much more skillful in reviewing the menu of opportunities, learning of the possibilities for gifting by this donor now and as well going forward in the future with other opportunities, and structuring the gifting arrangement so as to be maximally beneficial to the donor and to the Department/AHC.

i) It is exceedingly important for the Chair to realize that often the first gifting is a "trial balloon" by the donor. The smoother the process and the more reaffirming for the donor, the greater the possibility for subsequent gifts. These later gifts may be significantly larger, often in bequests in wills, trusts, and estates.

"Character may almost be called the most effective means of persuasion."

—ARISTOTLE

2) **Technology transfer, intellectual property, and patent revenues** are not historically traditional sources of revenue for academic Departments in AHCs. Some AHCs have been able to benefit from the proceeds of licensing and patents since the Bayh-Dole Act passed in 1980. AHCs have also espoused the principles of technology transfer in other ways besides licensing such as the sharing of research. In the past most AHCs have been less fortunate than those AHCs with the "big hits" from technology transfer and patents. Yet, ever hopeful, most AHCs do maintain and support an Office of Technology Transfer. These revenue opportunities may become more common with the increase in industry-AHC alliances (see chapters 29 and 32), and are an incredibly complex area. That said, the complexity well navigated with a great and marketable idea/product has the potential to be a very large source of Departmental and AHC incremental revenues. Vaccines are an excellent example. Think of the large sums of money accruing to those researchers and Departments that developed the vaccines for H. flu, for poliomyelitis, or for the HPV virus. Other examples would include the patents for antiviral drugs (HIV and HCV) or for warfarin. That said, such "big hits" are not common and not predictable. In trying to discern how to proceed with possible but unknown future successes, the Chair, the researchers, the Department, and the AHC must have sound legal and business advice. Often the AHC's in-house experts will suffice, but they may elect to contract out some of the particularly troublesome issues. These opportunities are deceptively complex, advice will be detailed, the process is surprisingly long, and the temptation to get frustrated is great. It is key to recognize that research brilliance and/or clinical expertise often leads to impatience and desires

to take shortcuts: "Can't you see how great this idea and product is, all the good that will come of it, and how much money might result? Let's just do it." This emotional statement by the academics who conceived the discovery is common, but it will be of little weight with those experts involved in the legal and business issues. Research and/or clinical brilliance does not translate to legal and business acumen (see chapters 20, 31, and 32).

One matter to be clearly delineated before any dollars are realized is the allocation of the revenues among the University (or the AHC), the Department, and the researcher (or researchers) involved. Once revenues start to accrue, it will be challenging to adjudicate the allocation of these monies to the AHC endowment, the Department endowment, current operating expenses, the faculty involved, or recruitment packages, etc.

3) **Start-up companies** can be lucrative but have many potential problems and pitfalls lurking for the enthusiastic faculty. The prudent Chair is aware of all of these issues, the need for legal and business input, and will actively mentor the faculty member(s) to be certain that all faculty involved, the Department, and the AHC have their interests protected and that there will be the greatest possible legitimate financial benefit.

One challenging issue for Chairs and the AHC is the conflict of commitment for the involved faculty in a start-up company. This does not just involve the relevant faculty but also the students and other trainees.

a) Research and/or clinical expertise may yield wonderful potential ideas, but research and/or clinical expertise and enthusiasm does not translate to business experience and acumen.

b) Faculty often do not appreciate the fatal flaw of venturing outside their skill sets, failing to obtain early and ongoing input from business experts.

c) New companies require "angel capital" investments by business and/or financial entrepreneurs for start-up money. The number of dollars required will be surprisingly large. Far more capital will be required than most medical academics appreciate. One matter to consider is that the involvement of the "angel investor" may be essential but will carry with it some loss of control of the direction of the start-up.

d) Should the AHC (and/or University) invest as some sort of co-owner providing initial capital? If so, institutional potential conflicts of interest must be identified and analyzed, and management plans developed. Issues are many and include commitment of AHC research resources for additional research in the scientific area(s) related to the start-up.

e) Developing sequential business plans takes much time and expertise. If full-time faculty propose a major role for themselves, it may pose time constraints incompatible with responsibilities of full-time faculty at AHC and create what is known as a conflict of commitment for those faculty members.

f) If the faculty believe their scientific involvement for input is essential in providing the key linkages between the science and the business, creative leaves of absence or part-time appointments may be required for the faculty.

g) The failure rate of start-ups is distressingly high, yet some start-ups may mature into a significant companies with their own stature. Others realize the maximum financial potential by being "bought out" early (purchased) by a much larger commercial enterprise. Sometimes the start-up will blossom into a full, mature company—and then often will be bought out by a much larger company. Either will result in major incremental revenues to the AHC, the Department, the researchers, and the angel funders.

h) The intellectual property issues are usually major.

i) Faculty must recognize and comply with the essential dictates from experts in patent law, intellectual property, finance, and conflict-of-interest management plans.

In spite of all these cautions, the combination of brilliant research, marketable products, astute business planning, prudent start-up financing, essential legal input for intellectual property and patents, and perseverance can result in gratifying start-up success. The results provide major revenue resources to the AHC, to the Department, to the involved faculty—and to the angel investors (see chapter 32 for considerations on conflict of interest).

4) **Relationships with industry** are important and have the potential to be much more so. AHCs possess creative engines yielding great science that may have major economic value going forward. That said, the AHC and the angel investors usually lack the enormous financial resources and skill sets available in industry. A "marriage" of AHCs and the pharmaceutical and device industries is a necessary and "good" development. These relationships take many forms, and require AHC input by Office of Counsel, Institutional Research Review Board, Office of Research Project Administration, Office of Technology Transfer, and the experts within the AHC responsible for developing conflict- of-interest management plans. The Chair must recognize the need to coordinate all of these inputs with the faculty and research involved in these commercial efforts.

> *"Why not go out on a limb? That's where the fruit is."*
> —WILL RODGERS

5) One emerging and complex relationship is occurring at the institutional level. As an example, a pharmaceutical or device industry grants or gifts many millions (to date, on occasion even hundreds of

millions) of dollars to a University or an AHC, in return for which intellectual and patent opportunities with eventual marketing revenues are linked to this arrangement. Controversies abound in this area. Issues involve, but are not limited to: academic freedom for the faculty involved in the research, timely publishing of results by the academician without industry censorship, and not permitting private-sector partners to license university intellectual property without plans to develop and commercialize it. The legal scope and conflict management issues are beyond the scope of this book, but Chairs need to be aware of these possibilities and work with the AHC's experts listed in the prior paragraphs to achieve the desired result.

Unrelated to these major institutional liaisons referenced in the preceding paragraphs, there are two specific potential relationships with industry for individual faculty members—**consulting and speakers' bureaus**. The Chair must be involved and mentor these faculty. Because of the dollars involved, discussions may become contentious. Although these AHC industry partnerships may often be desirable and can potentially advance the academic mission by generating new information, it is key to recognize that these relationships cannot be established under terms that will compromise ethics and the core AHC mission in research, which is to generate new knowledge for the public good. It is worth noting that this core mission requires open and rapid publication of research results, which can be contentious for industry.

1) **Consulting arrangements** need to be carefully vetted. These situations of mutual benefit to the faculty member and to the industry are important but have potential risks. Industrial research leaders need input from the AHC research and clinical leaders. What are the unsolved disease problems, what difficulties are being encountered with current medications and devices, what facets of faculty's research might have a bearing, and/or what clinical problems are occurring? Industry wants and needs this academic input. Matching

this, leading researchers and/or clinicians may need industrial connections to bridge the gap between their research drugs/devices and
product development/marketing. This can be win-win. That said,
there are "snakes in the grass," most of which will require conflict-
of-interest management plans (see also chapter 32). Issues include,
but are not limited to:

a) Is the faculty member permitted to do any research that is funded
directly by this company?

b) Is the faculty member permitted to do research, funded by
sources such as the NIH, on products made and marketed by
this company?

c) Are the consulting fees paid to the faculty member reasonable
for the time involved?

d) Has the consulting contract been vetted by the Office of Counsel
to be certain there are no problems with issues such as intellectual
property rights?

e) If indicated, are proper conflict-of-interest management plans in
place?

f) Are the conflict-of-management plans being followed?

g) Are all aspects of the consulting arrangement consistent with all
policies of the AHC and/or University?

2) **Speakers' bureaus** are a much more controversial matter for faculty participation. To be clear, the term "speakers' bureau" refers to
educational programs run by industry, marketed to clinicians, with
the educational speakers for those programs being academic faculty paid for by the company. These academic speakers' reputations
become an advertising tool for the company. There is often a fine
line of distinction between true education of the attendee physicians
versus marketing of the drug/device to attendees using the famous

academic speakers as salespeople. There is a big difference between continuing medical education within the guidelines of the ACCME given by accredited institutions and marketing presentations where faculty are salespeople for the company. Some of these "educational" programs can be in fancy restaurants or even resorts. These may present the opportunity for the company to provide unseemly lush perks to the speakers. Some companies even insist the speakers use only slides provided by the company; the companies use the reason that it is important that the speaker not advocate offline use of the drug/device and expose the company to unnecessarily risky liability. Most AHCs are now prohibiting faculty involvement in these industry events. For those AHCs that choose to permit faculty to participate in speakers' bureaus, most insist the faculty member use his/her own slides.

For the above reasons and complexities involved, many if not most AHCs do not permit faculty to participate in speakers' bureaus.

Be a Leader
Make a Difference
Enjoy!

CHAPTER 31

The Chair's Potpourri of Academic Challenges from Outside and Inside the AHC

> *"God, grant me the serenity to accept the things I cannot change; courage to change the things I can; and wisdom to know the difference."*
>
> —REINHOLD NIEBUHR (THE SERENITY PRAYER)

There are many other items in the Chair's potpourri of academic challenges. The list is ever expanding. At the time this was written, some of these were:

- Interfacing with and compliance with national accreditation, regulatory and/or funding bodies: Accreditation Council for Graduate Medical Education(ACGME), Accreditation Council for Continuing Medical Education (ACCME), Residency Review Committees (RRCs), Americal Board of Medical Specialties (ABMS), Joint Commission on Accreditation of Healthcare Organizations (JCAHO), National Institutes of Health (NIH), Medicare and HHS, etc.)

- Compliance with state and federal regulations, such as those of the NIH or those of HHS and HIPAA

- Challenges from labor laws and human resources

- The role of basic research in clinical Departments

- The role of fellowships in clinical Departments that have residencies

- Loss of funding for residencies and fellowships

- Seeking additional funding sources for medical school research and educational missions

- Issues of conflicts of interest and management thereof (institution, Departmental, and faculty)

- Issues of tenure and salary linkages

In this chapter, the author scans the landscape of broad-ranging challenges facing Department Chairs. The Chair acting alone in a vacuum will not solve these issues. Just as the issues are complex, the solutions are usually complex and are addressed by teams of individuals from the Chairs, the faculty, the administrators, compliance officials, the Office of Counsel, human resources, etc. Solutions are not suggested in this chapter but rather the challenges. Solutions will change, as the targets are moving. The Chairs must be involved; their leadership and team participation is essential if the AHC is to remain robust.

> *"If you don't know where you are going, you might not get there."*
> —YOGI BERRA

The Departmental activities that need to be managed by the Chair are becoming progressively more impacted and regulated by forces and regulatory bodies external to the Department, some originating outside the AHC on the national and state levels, some originating within the AHC. In many ways these regulatory probes interface to impact the Department. For example:

1) NIH policies on conflict of interest (COI) interface with and drive institutional policies and practices of COI reporting and management.

2) Changing government reimbursements for residency training inter-
sect with (and may compromise) the Department's attempts to comply with RRC and ACGME policies and regulations.

There are many national accreditation bodies external to the AHC
(ACGME, ACCME, RRC, ABMS, JCAHO, NIH, HIPAA). Interfacing
with these and compliance with all their regulations and policies is a
challenge and is compounded by state and federal regulations. All this
has become a very important and very time-consuming obligation
of academic Chairs. With the exception of the Liason Committee on
Medical Education (LCME) and the NIH, which impact all components
of the AHC, all of these listed organizations have the major direct impact on clinical Departments. That said, the basic science Chair needs
to be aware of these factors, as their impact may well impact adversely
the resources available in the AHC to support research and education.

Because of all the interfaces and interdigitations of these regulations
that impact Departments, separation into stand-alone topics is not realistic. Hence, these challenges for the Chair are grouped in clusters. The
author admits these clusters are arbitrary and are intended to focus on
the area(s) and mission(s) of the Department that are impacted.

1) **ACGME (Accreditation Council for Graduate Medical
   Education), ACCME (Accreditation Council for Continuing
   Medical Education), RRC (Residency Review Committees), ABMS
   (American Board of Medical Specialties)** are all organizations with
   real authority and power.

   a) The regulations and policies of each must be closely followed.
      Noncompliance can result in loss of residency programs and/
      or loss of credentialing authority for CME activities. The details
      and Departmental obligations of each are lengthy and complex,
      so much that the Departmental Chair will usually appoint a
      highly respected senior faculty member to lead the educational
      compliance efforts, and that faculty member will need full-time,

senior, experienced lay staff support. These two individuals will report to the Chair, as the Chair will retain the ultimate responsibility for compliance activities.

b) The role of fellowships in clinical Departments that have residencies is a discussion with many ramifications. There are basically two types of fellowships, and the Chair must decide how many, if any, will exist in the Department—and of what type.

   i) Fellowships accredited by the ACGME. Those that are accredited by the ACGME go through a process of evaluation and critique very similar to the stringency of that for residencies.

   ii) Fellowships that are not accredited are usually called "Departmental fellows." Those that are not accredited are in that category for one or more of several reasons, of varied merit. The five most common are:

   (1) The fellowship encompasses a very small defined area, with so few experts nationally, that although a legitimate area of study and training, the "market" is so limited as to not justify the national resources required by the ACGME to mount an accreditation process.

   (2) The fellowship is not accredited because the Department needs to bill for the fellow's services. With the constrictions in GME funding to hospitals by Medicare and other third-party payors and the resultant limitations on funded positions for residents and fellows, there are no institutional funds to support the fellowship. The ACGME precludes reimbursements for clinical care by a fellow in an accredited fellowship, even if the fellow is board-eligible. Hence, although the fellowship may be excellent, the fellowship director and the Department Chair have

had to decide to forgo accreditation in order to provide a billing source to support the fellowship position(s).

(3) The Departmental fellowship has little academic value and would never pass an ACGME accreditation visit.

(4) In some situations the number of fellows may create budget challenges for the Department (and for the AHC); in some occasions the number of fellows actually exceed the number of faculty (e.g., placed in expensive research programs).

(5) The Departmental fellowship is in place to provide board-eligible individuals to augment faculty clinical efforts. For example, all graduating chief residents are mandated to remain for an extra year of "trauma experience" as "junior faculty" covering the emergency room on a relatively low salary, with the Department billing for the resulting clinical services.

c) The Chair needs to understand and deal with the implications of fellowships for resident training. Does the presence of fellows enhance the resident educational experience, or do the fellows "get in the way" and diminish the resident experience? If the Department is well-balanced with all clinical areas of expertise, well staffed by fellowship-trained faculty, and with clinical volumes so large in each subspecialty area that residents cannot cover all the clinical activities in the clinics and in the operating rooms, the fellow is a welcomed addition. He/she can: a) share in the workload; b) enhance the teaching experience for the residents; and c) generally be involved in cases so advanced as to be beyond that of resident capabilities. In the contrary situation, the fellow intrudes and takes experience away from the resident education.

2) **Another cluster of external challenges is the lack of funding to provide resident training for adequate numbers of physicians in the**

future for the growing and aging US population. There is a projected need for more physicians; medical schools are responding by graduating more MDs and DOs, but there are not enough residency positions. Several years ago the federal government set quotas for the total number of residency trainees permitted in each AHC. These arbitrary quotas are already not adequate to cover the AHC costs to train current residents in training programs. These unreimbursed costs are a real debit to many AHCs with resultant financial burdens. The problem is becoming worse with the influx of more medical school graduates, as encouraged by this country's governments to meet the anticipated increase in need for physicians with the ever-aging population. More physicians will be needed, and challenges arise, including:

a) The Chair has to compete within his/her AHC for funded residency positions.

b) Resident hour restrictions result in the need for more residents to provide the service requirements and because of more limited resident experiences, may dictate the need for more years of residency training, especially in the procedural technical specialties.

c) There is some pressure to shorten the duration of residency training, with advancement through the residency to be based upon "competencies." This is worrisome for areas of training with great complexity, where large volumes of clinical experience are necessary for the trainee to have been exposed to and involved in the many subtle aspects. How can the Chair redesign the resident experience should this fundamental change be mandated? Does the AHC wish to unleash partially trained "specialists" who may well fail the ABMS certification processes and provide suboptimal care?

d) Physician assistants (PA) and/or nurse practitioners (NP) are being added to provide the service requirements by replacing residents who are now mandated to work fewer hours. The NP and PA are actually more expensive for Departments or the AHC, as unlike the residents, they do not work eighty hours a week. This is a funding challenge, to be negotiated between the Chair and the AHC.

e) As the capabilities have increased for more and more treatments that help patients, more care is being rendered, taking more faculty and resident effort. This poses increasing human-resource challenges.

f) The population is aging with a bolus of so-called "baby boomers," again increasing the demands for more physicians to be trained in the absence of funding to do so.

g) The Affordable Care Act will be infusing an estimated 30 million more patients into the system, already strained with inadequate number of physicians in many specialties.

h) Because of the intrusion of government regulations into the practice of medicine, many physicians are electing to retire early, rather than coping with these emerging issues.

> *"When you come to a fork in the road, take it."*
> —YOGI BERRA

> *"The most difficult thing is the decision to act; the rest is merely tenacity."*
> —AMELIA EARHART

3) **The government is changing policies on hospital reimbursement** that may well impact what training areas and specialties will be funded. Chairs of clinical Departments will need to get involved in the decisions as to the balance of training positions for primary care vs. specialty training.

a) How is primary care to be defined? Does this include just Family Medicine? Or does this include Obstetrics? Pediatrics? Internal Medicine?

b) Will the future model of primary care include relatively few MDs, with each supervising a cohort of NPs and/or PAs?

c) What will be the impact of "medical homes" and "population medicine"?

4) **LCME (Liaison Committee on Medical Education)** oversees the details of the medical school's educational programs, involving all aspects of the full curriculum and thus all basic science and clinical Departments. Similar to the ACGME for residencies, the LCME will conduct periodic on-site visits to the Medical School, and inadequate compliance with LCME regulations and guidelines will result in loss of medical school accreditation. With each passing year, more and more materials merit addition to the medical student curriculum. There is an ongoing transition in medical student education; students are being directed as adult learners, with much more emphasis on directed self-study in the medical schools' curricula. The Department Chair finds it progressively difficult to obtain adequate allocated curriculum time for several reasons. There is an exponential growth in information, yet much of what the student is expected to learn may prove to be erroneous in future years as knowledge increases from research progress. A powerful tool for emerging students, residents, and faculty is information technology with medical-library-assisted computer-based data searches for up-to-date information retrieval. This is expensive. What are the funding sources?

The Chair is challenged to gain or retain curriculum time, competing with other Chairs. The Chairs are facing the need for students to be taught to access knowledge based on computer access; but this is factual knowledge, not clinical skills. There is an increasing need for simulators, particularly expensive in robotics.

> *"A government big enough to give you everything
> you want is also strong enough to take everything
> you have."*
> —THOMAS JEFFERSON

5) HIPAA Regulations (Health Insurance Portability and Accountability Act), JCAHO (Joint Commission on Accreditation of Healthcare Organizations), ACA (Accountable Care Act) are all components of overarching national regulations, each impacting the AHC in its entirety. HIPAA regulations were initially put in place to protect patient privacy of medical information. It is well-intentioned; however, with the implementation of electronic medical records, the very beneficial result of access to patients' personal medical information across many sites for many providers results in major challenges to ensure patient privacy. The JCAHO, along with various state and federal agencies, do regular inspections of all health-care sites; failure to comply with standards will result in loss of licensure of the health-care sites and/or loss of authorization to bill third-party payors and/or Medicare/Medicaid programs. In addition, HIPAA issues can result in investigations by the Office of Civil Rights, followed by major fines.

6) **NIH regulations, policies, and systems are becoming more complex, at the same time as research grants are more difficult to obtain with the decreases in available federal research funding.** Layered on top of all the processes for grant funding are many new regulations for reporting to the federal government of information on all income sources to faculty that originate outside the AHC, with strict reporting requirements on industry funding (including travel, meals, etc.). The Chair has the responsibility for oversight for all such personnel in his/her Department. Other state and federal regulations are important, continually changing, and may vary from state to state. These involve institutional review boards, protection

of research subjects, biosafety, animal-use committees, and complex reporting obligations. All AHCs will have in-house expertise in these areas, and it is mandatory for each Chair to coordinate closely with those individuals as indicated by the specific situations.

7) **There are many regulatory bodies and policies within the AHC** that are driven by external forces and regulations from government. Interfacing with the government-mandated regulations and regulatory bodies within the AHC is an additional essential responsibility of the Chair. These AHC policies and committees impacting Departments and faculty include:

a) Clinical compliance areas, including: credentialing of faculty; licensure issues, and due diligence thereof; and clinical care documentation and billing compliance for clinical services. This latter is of immense complexity as the new ICD-10 coding contains thousands of choices, and billing regulations under ACA are in the thousands of pages.

b) Research activities must be in compliance with the Institutional Review Board and Research Administration policies, mostly mandated by federal agencies.

c) Conflict-of-interest management plans must be put in place as indicated and monitored. Driven by federal regulations, most AHC now will have a mandated yearly reporting of all outside income for all faculty to a centralized database at the AHC (see Chapter 32).

8) **Some factors external to the AHC are powerful economic forces impacting the research and educational budgets of AHCs.** Funding sources for medical schools is a significant challenge and this challenge will increase going forward. Even though tuition costs are very high for the individual student, even in state-funded medical schools, the tuition revenue falls far short of covering costs to the institution. In fact, tuition costs do not even provide the medical

school with sufficient funds to reimburse faculty for the time and effort to prepare for and deliver teaching exercises for the students, be those in lecture format or in smaller groups. Currently, most medical schools cobble together the necessary funds, in addition to tuition, from the following sources:

a) Endowments are an obvious source. However, in many AHCs the endowments have strict directions and guidelines from the donor as to how the revenues from that endowment gift are to be used. Most often, those funds are directed to support specific programs or research areas. A few schools have significant general endowment or even endowment specifically to fund medical student education.

b) Hospital revenues from some hospitals either owned by the University or with medical school affiliations have been able to direct funds from profit margins to augment medical school budgets. Unfortunately with the ACA and with decreasing hospital revenues combined with increasing costs for personnel (especially if unionized), hospitals are facing loss of margins, inability to fund necessary improvement and/or maintenance for equipment and facilities; and many hospitals are now in significant financial deficit.

c) Faculty clinical practice revenues, once also a source of some AHC revenue surplus to support education, are now facing financial restrictions. Just as for hospital clinical income, faculty practice income is no longer a funding source to supplement the costs of educational and research activities.

d) All of the preceding funding sources are changing with national and regional economic changes. All these changes are leading to austerity in almost all AHC and medical schools, with the very uncommon exception of the highly endowed institutions with endowments targeted for education and for research.

9) **Issues of tenure and salary guarantees are becoming increasingly important**, and the options available to the AHC and the Departmental Chairs are complex, restrictive, and driven by state and federal laws in human resources and by employment contract law. Historically, academic tenure has been highly valued by faculty. Tenure is an honor bestowed in acknowledgement of academic success and is granted by the AHC and the University in expectation of continued academic prowess and success. That said, another reason tenure appointments are so important to those faculty so honored is that tenure has implied a certain level of salary guarantee. This so-called "guarantee" varies from AHC to AHC and is often very disparate between clinical Departments and basic science Departments. In some undergraduate schools, the academic institution "guarantees" the entire salary. In AHCs, the guarantee for clinicians may be only a few thousand dollars each year but for basic scientists "the guarantee" can be a significant percentage of the total salary. Definite difficulties due to these disparities are occurring for several understandable and predictable reasons. The possible solutions are made more complex by legal and human resource mandates originating external to the Department, as the AHC in turn is responding to the external forces of state and federal law.

a) The previously mandated AHC and University faculty retirements at age sixty-five are now illegal under federal law for reasons of "age discrimination." Thus, the AHC and the University are now faced with expanding financial commitments to older faculty.

b) The presence of faculty who "hang on" beyond productive years tie up academic monies with their salaries, precluding the hiring of new, young faculty early in their career (see chapter 26, 28).

c) University and AHC endowments are usually not enough to cover these obligations.

290

d) Universities and AHCs are struggling to cope with marked decreases in external funding from government research grants and from third-party payors for health-care reimbursements. Thus, it is no longer realistic for AHCs to "guarantee" salary for nonproductive faculty, even for those with tenure. There is the resultant need for AHCs to have detailed and clear faculty-compensation plans for all faculty (clinical and research) that are linked to productivity.

e) The potential solutions are many, complex, and must be carefully designed and implemented specific to the AHC and state, with solid advice and input from the Office of Counsel. Initial offer letters, all reappointment letters, and all correspondence at the time faculty are considered for tenure must contain language explaining that salaries can increase or decrease depending upon faculty productivity and AHC/University finances. Ideally the term *guarantee* will not be used in these documents, but rather language such as, "Your salary for this year will be $X, paid monthly in twelve equal amounts. In addition you may qualify for salary bonus of $Y based upon your productivity defined as XXXX and ZZZZ. This incremental salary will be paid (monthly, quarterly). Future salary levels will be determined yearly and may be adjusted as necessary based upon productivity metrics as outlined in the faculty practice plan." (see chapters 26, 27, and 28; appendices A, B, C))

f) Labor law and human-resource issues are complex, not only for faculty, but for all staff and employees. Unfortunately, these complexities are ever increasing. They impact the faculty, the residents, and the staff in the Department.

　　i) Complexities involve significant variability and differences—hourly vs. salaried, union vs. nonunion, design of benefit plans, implication of "salary bands" in benefit-cost allocations, diversity definitions and policies, reporting responsibilities to governments, etc.

ii) Human-resource and labor law is now a subspecialty area, and Senior Leadership, Chairs, and Center/Program directors must solicit and follow this legal advice.

iii) Logic and common sense may be irrelevant, but compliance with the laws in this area is mandatory. The hours spent initially in doing things properly are well invested, and far less time-consuming and much less expensive than the time and expenses required to unravel earlier inadvertent decisions.

> *" When everything seems to be going against you, remember that the airplane takes off against the wind, not with it."*
> —Henry Ford

. . . .

Be a Leader
Make a Difference
Enjoy!

. . . .

CHAPTER 32

Evolving Basic, Clinical, and Translational Research; Emergence of Conflict of Interest—Implications and Challenges

> "A clever person turns great troubles into little ones
> and little ones into none at all."
> —CHINESE PROVERB

Many areas of basic science, such as vaccine biology or immunology, have such clinical relevance that linkages are and should be evolving with clinical Departments. Many clinical Departments with MD/PhD clinical scientists bring basic science disciplines and insights to clinical problems they confront. Both of these basic science and clinical Department situations foster increasingly productive translational research. But the road may not be smooth, with challenges to be recognized and solved.

Most AHCs today are prioritizing research efforts and linkages to foster research that moves from bench to bedside, and from bedside back to bench, within a translational framework. Departments that have this capacity, either within that Department or by collaborations across the AHC, will emerge to a winning favorable position within the AHC.

Basic research in clinical Departments can have great value and relevance, but relationships with basic science Departments and promotion systems need to be delineated and coordinated.

1) Advantages are several for doing basic science in clinical Departments, and perhaps the greatest is the fostering of the clinician scientist with one foot in clinical care and the other foot firmly planted in NIH-funded basic science. This duality of expertise tremendously augments the translational clinical relevance of the research—basic science brought to the bedside, and equally important, unsolved clinical problems brought to the research bench. The PhD scientists working so closely with the clinician scientist can benefit from his/her insights and at the same time, broaden the spectrum of research projects in the Department.

2) Funding source implications in these arrangements can be several. First, with the NIH-funding line changes and the increasing emphasis in translational research in federal funding and industry-funding sources, the potential advantages for successful grant applications are obvious. During times of diminished extramural funding between grants, the opportunities for philanthropy in clinical Departments and/or use of some clinical academic revenues to sustain research are significant, important, and challenging.

3) The situation as viewed by basic research Departments is important to consider. Understandably, robust basic science programs in clinical Departments may not be well received by basic science Departments, which may feel threatened. There are some proactive steps that can be very helpful.

   a) Be certain that teaching obligations for medical students and PhD candidates are the same for all basic scientists, whether that individual's primary appointment is in a clinical or basic science Department.

   b) Be certain that the criteria for promotion of those faculty doing basic science research is the same, regardless of the location of the faculty member's primary academic appointment.

"A beautiful thing is never perfect."
— EGYPTIAN PROVERB

There are several **reasons to increase linkages across Departments, Centers, and Programs.**

1) Excellent faculty members with meaningful productive interdigitations across several Departments and with resultant dual appointments will usually be more successful with grant funding in the era of research complexity.

2) Such multi-Departmental arrangements with key collaborators may be very difficult to replicate in another AHC, enhancing retention of such excellent faculty.

3) These arrangements can make a very positive impact on decreasing the "silo mentality" that traditionally has been so prevalent and is now so detrimental.

4) Funding agencies are increasingly looking to interdisciplinary research models. Therefore, an AHC's promotion and tenure system for faculty needs to evolve to support such interdisciplinary research for such highly collaborative faculty who have expert coinvestigator input roles on multiple research projects, although not the PIs on any of these projects as "their own." Promotion systems in AHCs need to recognize the co-PI legitimacy for all faculty with substantial involvement.

The increasing role, relevance, and funding for translational research is important.

1) Translational research relates well with the activity in clinical Departments but not exclusively so, as many basic scientists have research that has real clinical relevance.

2) Funding opportunities are many, not only for grant funding, but also:

a) Patent and intellectual property opportunities

b) Relationships with industry with AHC-industry alliances—both device and pharmaceutical companies. These industries' interest and increasing involvement are becoming an important reality with many contract opportunities of great value to future patient care, to the AHC research programs, and to the commercial industries (see also chapters 29 and 30). The public-private partnerships being promoted by NIH (especially via the CTSA programs) are of significant importance.

c) There are other government programs targeting research to improve and develop higher-quality health care with cost controls.

d) Many of these funding opportunities carry with them the need to accurately identify and properly manage conflicts of interest.

> *"My destination is no longer a place, rather a new way of seeing."*
> —MARCEL PROUST

This evolving basic, clinical, and translational research can become an institutional strength or conversely, can be a detrimental force codifying the silo mentality. With the emergence of excellent basic science in clinical Departments and research with immediate clinical relevance in basic science Departments, conflicts and tensions will arise, real or perceived, between the basic science and clinical Departments. The basic science Department and faculty may resent and belittle basic research prospering in clinical Departments. Conversely, clinicians may resent basic research emerging into clinical areas—such as vaccines developed in a basic science Department perceived as intruding on the turf of clinical infectious disease experts. Chairs and Senior Leadership need to be very proactive to foster a collaborative atmosphere, with "Centers of Excellence" concepts rather than silos.

Financial conflicts of interest (COI) situations are a reality and management is essential.

> *"Rocks in my path? I keep them all. With them I shall build my castle."*
> —Nemo Nox

The conflict of interest that is attracting much national interest, both in the lay press and especially in the federal government, is financial conflict of interest (COI) (see also chapter 30).

1) These are the situations involving the real economic and potential economic benefits accruing to the faculty, the Departments, the AHC, and the University. These economic benefits are the result of:

   a) Linkages with industry for product development, clinical trials, and then marketing

   b) Grants and gifts from industry to AHCs

   c) Intellectual property, technology transfer

   d) Awarding of patents (now or potential)

   e) Start-up company endeavors (already under way or even just in the conceptual stage)

2) In brief, the conflict, real or perceived, occurs when the objectivity of research results might be compromised, or perceived to be potentially compromised, by the opportunity to alter research results to enhance the revenues coming from the business and/or patent and/

or intellectual property to the AHC, the Department, or a faculty member.

3) The design of adequate, realistic, and prudent management plans requires several steps.

a) Some confidential mechanism must exist within the AHC for faculty to disclose all sources of outside financial assets and income going to him/her and to family from sources external to the AHC that relate to his/her AHC work. These outside financial assets are defined broadly to include contracts, consulting fees, speaker fees, stocks, stock options, fiduciary roles, and any intellectual property involving or created external to the AHC. These disclosures should be done on a yearly basis, and within a defined period should new sources of outside income arise during the course of the year between the annual disclosures. Upgrades during the year are necessary if situations change. A confidential web-based question form is extraordinarily helpful in tabulating information, analyzing data, developing management, and tracking compliance with management plans.

b) Some group of knowledgeable individuals outside the Department or Center should review all the disclosures as made and develop a list of faculty from whom more information is needed.

c) Once the additional information is obtained, the materials are presented and discussed by a key knowledgeable group, decisions made as to which faculty require management plans, and then the management plan is created.

d) All of this disclosure and reporting information, including the management-need decisions and the resultant management plans for the potential conflict of interest, must be in compliance with PHS requirements for investigators funded by PHS/NIH grants.

e) Suggested composition of the preceding described group:

    i) Ideally is chaired by a senior faculty member from the Dean's Office to provide the necessary authority linkage to Senior Leadership

    ii) Includes senior representatives from the Office of Counsel, the Office of Research Projects Administration, and the Institutional Review Board

    iii) Includes enough senior faculty to constitute at least half the total group membership: senior faculty here is defined as "old enough to be wise, and young enough to be alert," Professor level, and known to possess institutional vision rather than parochial interests

f) The group, via the Dean's Office reporting connection, must have the support of the Dean and CEO, including withdrawal of institutional support and resources from faculty who refuse to cooperate with this COI management system.

g) Reporting from this group should go via the Dean to the CEO of the AHC, and thence to the Provost and President of the University should that be the organizational institutional structure.

4) COI can occur within AHCs in many forms, and a few examples follow. Note that COI is such a complex area with so many variances and combinations that, "Once you've seen one COI that needs to be managed, you've seen one."

a) Institutional COI:

    i) The AHC has an equity position in a start-up company, emerging from the research work of a faculty member. Additional research is ongoing in that same area that spawned the new company and is being done by that same faculty member, along with several other faculty members and support staff. This research and resultant intellectual property will enhance the value and success of the start-up and the patents. The AHC leadership has to decide to whom to allocate additional research resources within the institution—the group connected to the start-up or other research labs at the AHC? And, in addition, the Dean has requested permission to sit on the managing board of this new company.

ii) The CEO of the AHC has been asked to become a director of a large company. The AHC purchases significant supplies from that company.

b) Departmental COI:

i) A great deal of research on "Super Stuff" is being conducted in a specific academic Department, "Wow." This research is funded by NIH grants. The research is being done by faculty member "I. M. Good." The Wow Department Chair's own academic research is in "Hot Stuff," funded in part by "Too Hot." The Chair of the Wow Department has to decide allocation of lab space and hard-money support between research projects Super Stuff and Hot Stuff. These conflicts are compounded because the spouse of the Chair of the Wow Department has an appointment in another academic Department, and is a consultant for company Too Hot and is speaking to other spouses in the Wow Department about buying stock in Too Hot.

ii) A faculty member is a part owner of a start-up company and asks the Department Chair to invest in the company.

c) Individual faculty COI:

 i) A faculty member with a robust research program has NIH grant funding in an area of research "A." This research involves several clinical trials of new drugs on human subjects. This research is in a focused area with very few recognized national leaders other than this faculty member. Because of this faculty member's recognized expertise, he/she has been asked to serve as a consultant for the company that makes these drugs.

 ii) A faculty member owns stock in company S. He/she is doing research with NIH funding and wants to be part of a multicenter clinical trial to study the clinical benefits of a drug marketed by company S.

Be a Leader
Make a Difference
Enjoy!

CHAPTER 33

The When and How for the Established Chair to Step Aside

> *"I have learned that success is to be measured not so much by the position that one has reached in life, as by the obstacles which he has overcome while trying to succeed."*
>
> —BOOKER T. WASHINGTON

The important aspects of this chapter make the assumptions that both the leader and the Department are doing well, or may even be exceeding all realistic expectations for success. The leader is still being successful in the current role as Chair. The Chair is not being asked to stop prematurely because of perceived poor performance.

There are several reasons a Chair may choose to step aside. This Chair has enjoyed being successful in that role for several years and he/she:

1) Is getting tired

2) Has a new health issue that precludes the effort and level of performance ideal for the leadership role

3) Has increasing family issues/responsibilities that divert much of the leader's time and energy and are projected to be long-term, not short-term

4) Has a fundamental difference in the direction(s) in which Senior Leadership is taking the AHC, that although honorable, are not

LEADING DEPARTMENT EXCELLENCE

those values or visions the Chair espouses, and hence, cannot in good faith be an enthusiastic leader within that environment

5) Is aware that new leadership is necessary to move the Department forward to the next level

6) The Chair, because of great successes, is being asked to assume a greater role at the AHC, such as to become the Dean or the AHC's CEO.

One other factor may be that the AHC has a policy of term limits for Chairs, even if the Chair has been and continues to be very effective.

> *"I don't want a country like ours to be led by an octogenarian. I must step down while there are one or two people who admire me."*
> —NELSON MANDELA

In this amicable situation, some suggested steps for this leader:

1) Proactively advise Senior Leadership of the desire to step aside, and with them decide on a time mutually optimal.

2) Work out a transition plan for a new Chair.

3) Agree with Senior Leadership as to whether the Chair should remain as Chair during the search, or step aside sooner and have an interim/acting Chair.

4) Offer to help with the search process by suggesting:

   a) Current faculty who would make an excellent successor as Chair

   b) Names he/she knows nationally who would be strong external candidates for Chair

c) National academic leaders who would be excellent external consultants to review the Department and make suggestions as to strengths, weaknesses, and opportunities for the Department that will be of aid to the search committee

5) Review the names of AHC faculty leaders and others from senior administration who would be prudent members of a search committee.

> *"If you get to thinking you're a person of some influence, try ordering somebody else's dog around."*
> —AUTHOR UNKNOWN

Obviously there are times when a Chair steps aside, and it is not his/her choice. There are many scenarios how this may occur, rarely pleasant. These situations usually are one of the following:

1) The AHC makes major organizational changes, and the Chair's position is eliminated. Such may occur when two Departments are combined to a single Department for reasons of evolving science, changes in patterns of clinical care, institutional efficiency, and/or institutional financial restraints.

2) The Chair's personal administrative, research, clinical, and/or style performance fall short of expectations. The Chair's Department functions poorly. This may occur within the first year of being Chair, after several years of declining results, or precipitated by a rapid sudden deterioration of the Department.

> *"Inside every older person is a younger person wondering what happened."*
> —TERRY PRATCHETT

When this type of situation occurs, the issues are contentious and controversial, and may often involve legal interventions. As these issues are driven by the individual situation, the comments are brief. Simply stated, the needs, goals, visions, and leadership of the AHC take precedence; the Chair had best accept the decision of the AHC and move on.

It is essential to recognize that the administrative appointment as Chair is separate from the academic appointment. The administrative appointment is at the pleasure of Senior Leadership, and thus can be terminated midappointment, providing the offer letter of the Chair position stipulated the distinction between the academic and administrative positions. That academic appointment may have been made with or without tenure.

The nontenure appointment has a time limit. Termination of tenure can be difficult, and this will usually involve some sort of financial settlement, negotiated by attorneys for the AHC and for the Chair who has been requested to leave.

> *"Sorrow looks back, Worry looks around, Faith looks up."*
> —RALPH WALDO EMERSON

CHAPTER 34
Life after Relinquishing Chair Leadership

> *"Some people try to turn back their odometers. Not me. I want people to know 'why' I look this way. I've traveled a long way and some of the roads weren't paved."*
>
> —WILL ROGERS

Those who have been prudent in Chair leadership positions will have already considered and planned for what is to be next for them in life's activities. Obviously that situation is much smoother to accomplish if the stepping-aside decision was initiated by the Chair and not the AHC.

Unfortunately, there are occasions when the AHC makes the decision and imposes the loss of the leadership position. If for cause, this may be with a rather short timeline. Although those in leadership Chair positions usually have tenure, the tenure is for the academic appointment, and not for the Chair or other leadership positions. Chair positions serve at the pleasure of the Dean or CEO.

> *"My destination is no longer a place, rather a new way of seeing."*
>
> —MARCEL PROUST

Whether the Chair's departure is planned or unanticipated, life can and should be meaningful for the former Chair leader. A couple of observations are obvious but merit listing:

1) Most Chairs and similar leaders achieved those positions by very hard work, dedication, and long hours focused on activities other than recreation and family. Those basic personality drives will continue into the new situation (35).

2) The new Chair leader often may take the Department in a new direction. This may be in conjunction with changes in Senior Leadership personnel and/or mission vision. The former Chair should be available if the new Chair seeks advice but otherwise should fade into the background.

3) Although an initial period of decompression, relaxation, etc., will be welcome, that welcome will be time-limited.

4) The ex-Chair needs a purpose to get up in the morning. Without some meaningful, directed activity, the former Chair may encounter a new stress, the stress of "I have no value or use." This may set the stage for major problems, such as depression, substance abuse, or other untoward behaviors.

5) The ex-Chair needs a new identity (35). The title under the name on the business card and under the name on the e-mail is no longer "Chair." What will it be? What is the new identity? Or will it be "Emeritus?"

6) Are there significant research, teaching, or clinical skills that the former Chair may choose to continue or resume in his/her new role?

7) Are there activities that the ex-Chair wishes he/she had done in years past but was always too busy? Now is the time to plan these.

8) The ex-Chair will need to develop new relationships, be those in volunteer organizations, at a health club, with peers who have similar hobbies, and/or in church activities.

9) Those ex-Chairs who had outside interests while in the Chair's leadership role are much better positioned for the transition to the new role.

10) Regardless of the above:

a) Proactively develop a bucket list of items that need attention in family, home, and personal life.

b) Plan some fun activities with family or friends totally unrelated to the former activities as Chair.

c) Enjoy each day.

d) Carefully review personal and family finances and retirement financial strategies.

e) Be certain financial planners, accountants, and estate planners are current, including power of attorney, wills, trusts (if any), medical advance-care directives, and authorization forms for someone else to make medical decisions should the former Chair be unable to do so personally.

> *"No memory of having starred*
> *Atones for later disregard*
> *Or keeps the end from being hard."*
> —ROBERT FROST

Regardless of any of the preceding variables, the situation now facing the former Chair presents many opportunities and positive challenges. Choices for the former Chair entering a new phase in life are many.

Schlossberg has some interesting insights on varous different approaches taken by individuals (32, 33) and describes:

1) Continue to use existing skills and interests.

2) Embark as an adventure on new endeavors with purposeful direction (35).

3) Search by trial and error, exploring new possibilities.

4) Glide along, letting each day happen with the leisure of unscheduled time.

5) Remain engaged in big issues as a spectator with some, but limited involvement, rather than being a driving force.

6) Retreat into a quiet disengagement.

As a former Chair and former Senior Associate Dean, this author has observed all of the above, and in fact has noted that individual former Chairs may well change approaches and styles with time. Any one of these can become a major interest, although most former Chairs will evolve to a combination of two or more, including, but not limited to, the following examples:

1) Those who expand the hobbies/activities of the "prior life" into a major interest, perhaps even a business.

    a) A former Chair with a genuine knowledge of furniture and who dabbled in woodworking, after stepping away from leadership and a surgical career, started making furniture for children and grandchildren. Soon this expanded as he was asked to make items for friends as "a favor" for gifts. Gradually this became a small business endeavor.

    b) A former Chair, once retired, became an expert in computer programming, even returning to school to learn new relevant skills.

> *"You cannot do a kindness too soon, for you never know how soon it will be too late."*
> —Ralph Waldo Emerson

2) Those who pick up a skill or talent from many years ago, update the training and emerge into a new career.

a) A Chair, years before in youth and college, had set aside a musical instrument to pursue a career in medicine. Once no longer a Chair, he enrolled in some performance courses and has now emerged into a modest symphony-performance career.

b) A Chair years before had dabbled in art. After stepping aside, he took lessons and became an accomplished landscape artist.

3) Some have transitioned a talent necessary in the prior role into a burst of related activity.

a) A former Chair, who in that role wrote many professional articles and edited some professional books, utilized those talents and connections to write and publish books on nonmedical topics of interest to him.

b) A former Chair, well published, became editor in chief of a major medical journal.

> *"No man ever steps in the same river twice, for it's not the same river and he's not the same man."*
> —Heraclitus

4) Former Chairs who look to one aspect of the former professional career, which was dwarfed by the leadership commitments, and resume a productive career in that rejuvenated role.

c) A former Chair with a very productive earlier research career that was crowded out by the time and responsibilities of being a Chair, took a sabbatical to rejuvenate some research skills, and upon return in a new role of "just research" had a very successful rewarding "life after Chair."

d) A former Chair in a primary care area volunteers much time, skill, and effort to care of the indigent via AHC clinics and outreach clinics via churches.

5) Others have taken up an entire new activity that had always been of intriguing curiosity, but the pressures of being Chair precluded any involvement—such as sitting on national or community charity boards, or becoming involved in volunteer activities such as Habitat for Humanity, food cupboards, Meals on Wheels.

6) A Chair with particular successes as a leader, or in a clinical/research and/or educational role, after stepping aside assumes a new role in the AHC mentoring others or nurturing programs in research/education/clinical area(s).

> *"Live simply. Love generously. Care deeply. Speak kindly. Leave the rest to God."*
> —Ronald Reagan

SECTION VI

Case Studies

The author is presenting these case studies as a separate section of the text, as each case study calls on skill sets and materials from several chapters. Each of these hypothetical scenarios presents dilemmas and challenges, similar to those occurring at many AHCs. Several of these cases have more than one problematic situation, these challenges often interfacing as solutions are sought. Each of these cases has no easy answers, as indeed is the situation in real life. In each of these, the Chair is pushed outside the normal MD and/or PhD medical skill sets, again as is what actually happens.

Should this book be used as a text for leadership development courses within an AHC, the author intends for these cases to be used to stimulate discussion in small group settings. Should the individual faculty member turn to this volume for personal development, these cases will hopefully serve to focus his/her thoughts in applying facts to foster function.

In approaching each case as the reader seeks solution(s), he/she is challenged to explore and consider:

1) What are *all* the key questions, essential facts, and less important aspects of the case? How many issues and problems are there?

2) What additional information and/or further facts are not in the case as presented, but which are necessary to know?

3) Where, how, and from whom can that information be learned or deduced?

4) Who are the key players in the case as presented?

5) Who are all the true stakeholders mentioned in the case as presented? Are there other stakeholders who might already have, or most likely will have in the future, a role in this case?

6) How should these stakeholders be involved in gathering information and creating strategies and solutions?

7) To whom in the AHC might the Chair turn for a sounding board, advice, or help?

8) Is the scenario a matter of ethics, financial issues, compliance with policies, harassment, diversity, criminal activity, research integrity—or a combination, and if so, what are all the elements?

9) What additional skill sets, which the leader may not possess, are needed to sort through the case?

10) Where might those skill sets be obtained, from inside or outside the AHC? At what cost? Who should pay for those costs?

11) From whom around the AHC might key resources and input be solicited and realistically expected?

12) Consider there may be more than one prudent course of action, and if so, what are the alternatives, which is better, and what are the reasons for that?

13) Who around the AHC might benefit if the Chair/leader fails to solve the situation? Does (do) that individual (those individuals) have the potential to influence adversely the outcome? If so, how

might that be neutralized, or even turned to advantage in this or other future similar scenarios?

14) What specific goal or result should the leader seek in solving the problem(s) presented in the case?

15) Of the solutions proposed by the Chair, what are possible adverse outcomes if the action(s) taken are not successful? What are the second-order possible solutions for the adverse outcome(s)?

16) In the proposed specific realistic strategic solution, a) what are the specific sequential steps; b) what is/are the desired outcome(s) and solution(s); and c) how will the result be "measured" as successful (i.e., a little successful, very successful, or unable to measure success)?

In the preceding sixteen guidelines for discussion and consideration, the reader must remember that in the big picture:

1) Stick to facts.

2) No emotion should show (especially anger or bitterness); this can be very hard in real-life situations.

3) Seek allies to make a win-win solution and strategy to achieve the goal(s).

Case 1:

A recently promoted Associate Professor, I. M. Smart, twenty-four months into her five-year appointment on an academic track, has just received her second NIH grant. She has several staff helping with her projects, one of whom is a young, single, male Research Instructor, Dr. Tester. Dr. Smart and her staff (especially Dr. Tester) work long hours, often extending well into the evenings. A female Research Instructor, Dr. I. M. Running, is uncomfortable as Dr. Tester is allegedly singled out by Dr. Smart for the better aspects of the project work, instead of Dr. Running. The disgruntled Dr. Running comes to the Chair, quite concerned that Dr. Smart is out of town from late Thursday afternoon until late on Monday almost all weekends, and in addition, takes one week a month to allegedly go to meetings. Upon questioning by the Chair, the disgruntled female Dr. Running admits that she looked at Dr. Smart's computer without permission (was not password-protected), suspecting an improper relationship of Dr. Smart with Dr. Tester, only to uncover e-mail exchanges of Dr. Smart with another AHC. Dr. Running states that these emails indicate that Dr. Smart also has a full-time salaried academic appointment at this other AHC.

Case 2:

An established midcareer male Associate Professor of Medicine with Tenure, Dr. I. Care, with a subspecialty in intensive care, has a series of personal medical problems for which several excellent colleague physicians are treating him. One of these conditions is a very painful diabetic neuropathy. A resident trainee, Dr. I. V. Drip, has been assigned to the ICU to work with Dr. Care, and she received poor performance reviews from Dr. Care. The residency Program Director, Dr. Busy, after reading the poor performance reviews of Dr. Drip, meets with her to discuss her performance and need for improvement. She is very upset and leaves his office in tears. Dr. Busy does not follow up Dr. Drip; she a few weeks later bypasses the Program Director and makes an appointment with the Chair, Dr. Charge. At that time, Dr. Drip accuses Dr. Care of being impaired by overuse of pain medications, including Oxycontin. The Chair to this point in time has not been aware of any quality-of-care issues by Dr. Care, and Dr. Busy has not spoken with Dr. Charge about Dr. Drip's performance reviews. The Chair's wife is an attorney specializing in wills and trusts at a large local law firm; she advises her husband to be cautious because the Americans with Disabilities Act may be applicable.

Case 3:

Dr. I. B. Shooter, the Chair of a large Department with many residents, both male and female, becomes aware of the following situation. One of the female chief residents, Dr. Capable, is having a sexual relationship with a male second-year resident, Dr. New, who is assigned to Dr. Capable's ward team. Dr. Capable is married to a third-year resident, Dr. I. B. Clueless, in another academic Department at the same AHC. Dr. New is married to a fourth-year medical student. The Chair meets with Dr. Capable, who does not deny the situation.

Case 4:

Non-tenured Associate Professor, Dr. Awesome, requests to meet with the Chair of the basic science Department, Dr. Super, in which Dr. Awesome has his primary academic appointment. Dr. Awesome is working on his own independent and NIH-funded research, but his area of independent research overlaps with the heavily funded (NIH and DoD) research of tenured full Professor, Dr. Hustle, in that same academic Department. Not only is Dr. Hustle a tenured Professor, but he holds a heavily endowed Chair. Both Dr. Awesome and Dr. Hustle have independent research space but do share some common space and resources. Both Dr. Awesome and Dr. Hustle have PhD candidates, I. Try and Will Fetch, working on research studies in the labs of Dr. Awesome and Dr. Hustle, respectively. Fetch comes to Try very upset about a situation evolving in the lab of Dr. Hustle, and with Try's urging, Fetch goes to speak with Dr. Awesome and to seek his advice. Dr. Awesome is very concerned about what he is told, and hence the meeting of Dr. Awesome with the Chair, Dr. Super. Dr. Awesome relates the following. Endowed Professor Hustle consults with a pharmaceutical company. The research project of Fetch in Professor Hustle's lab involves some drug structures very similar to those of a drug the pharmaceutical company is bringing to market, currently undergoing phase III trials; this early research of Fetch shows some major adverse effects in lab mice. Dr. Hustle is aware of this and is taking Dr. Fetch off that research project because "it shows no promise." Fetch is early into the research and Dr. Hustle is giving Fetch another project "that is better for you." The Chair promptly consults the computerized conflict-of-interest database of the AHC and learns that Professor Dr. Hustle received $100,000 total in cash, in addition to some stock, over the past two years for consultation with the pharmaceutical company. Furthermore, Professor Dr. Hustle has a signed contract with that pharmaceutical company. Fortunately, there is a copy of that contract in the faculty file of Professor Hustle in the Chair's office. The Chair reads it and discovers there is some language in that contract referencing "intellectual property rights." The language is legal and confusing to the Chair; the Chair is not certain what and whose intellectual property is referenced, just Dr. Hustle's or possibly extending to others in the AHC. In view of the results of the intellectual property litigation in other states, the Chair is concerned about this, as well as conflict-of-interest issues. As best the Chair can ascertain from the faculty files, this contract was never vetted by the AHC's Office of Counsel.

Case 5:

Dr. I. M. Trying has just become Chair of a busy clinical Department that has significant basic science activity. This Department does many procedures, mostly inpatient. The proper care of these inpatients generated many reimbursed services for several other clinical Departments and also for clinical hospital-based areas in the hospital. Thus, this clinical Department not only generates significant revenues for itself, but also for the hospital and for several other clinical Departments. A few months after becoming Chair, Dr. Trying receives a request to meet with the Chair of another Department, Dr. Compete, and the charge nurse of the operating room suite. At this meeting, Dr. Compete and the charge nursing supervisor express concerns about surgery being done by one of Dr. Trying's busiest surgeons, Dr. Slice. With further questioning, Dr. Compete and the nurse admit the surgery is being done well, but their major concerns are a) questionable indications for many of the procedures; and b) conversations they've both overheard suggesting issues of upcoding as well. The areas of clinical interest of Dr. Compete and Dr. Slice overlap. Dr. Trying's primary career focus is basic research.

Case 6:

Tenured Professor Established makes an appointment with her Chair, Dr. Wise, of basic science Department Mice. Professor Established is very upset and alleges that some of her lab data have been stolen, along with genetically engineered mice that she is using to conduct NIH-funded research. The Chair asks for more details, and Professor Established relates the following details. She has a relatively young laboratory technician, Ms. Do Good, who is good friends with another lab technician, Ms. Sneak, who works in another lab in Department Rats. Ms. Good looks up to Ms. Sneak, much as a younger sibling looks up to an older sibling. There is a well-funded tenured Associate Professor, Dr. Aggressive, in Department Rats, and Ms. Sneak works in one of the labs in Department Rats. Dr. Aggressive goes to Ms. Sneak and tells her that Professor Established has given him permission to use data and mice from Professor Establish's lab to help start a new research project for more grant funding. Dr. Aggressive asks Ms. Sneak to get those data and mice from friend Ms. Good. Ms. Sneak does this; Ms. Good complies. Professor Established becomes aware of this and is furious as she never gave the alleged permission.

Case 7:

Dr. Newbie, a recently appointed Chair of Department Good, has spent much time and effort getting to know each faculty member and his/her career aspirations, and thus the Chair is beginning to build consensus for developing a vision with a strategic plan for Department Good. Dr. I. Cut and Dr. Me Sew, two tenured Professors, are each very well-trained surgeons in highly subspecialized clinical fields (blood and guts). Both are well respected and well connected nationally. Dr. Cut is the only faculty member with subspecialty training in blood, and similarly Dr. Sew the only faculty member with subspecialty training in guts. The revenues from blood and guts are responsible for 70 percent of the clinical revenues for the Department. The reasons for this are not from lack of effort of other faculty and RVU effort of other faculty generating less revenue, but rather are payor-mix variations and inequalities in reimbursements for procedures performed. Although Drs. Cut and Sew express support of Dr. Newbie when face-to-face with this new Chair, Dr. Newbie is becoming distressingly aware that Drs. Cut and Sew are spreading false rumors about Dr. Newbie and the Department's planning, not only among other faculty within the Department but elsewhere in the AHC, such as in the operating rooms and clinics, in front of nurses and residents. Dr. Newbie begins to hear of similar rumors about himself from friends of his at other AHCs across the country. In the middle of these destabilizing events, a resident, Dr. Hopeful, who is dating one of last year's graduates from fellowship in blood, Dr. U Coming, who is now a new faculty in Department Good) makes an appointment with Dr. Newbie, at which Dr. Hopeful accuses Dr. Cut of falsifying an operative note and operative consent form. The Chair begins to look into that charge, and just two weeks later the Chair learns that Dr. Sew has interviewed for a professorial appointment at another AHC.

Case 8:

Dr. Basic is Chair of a well-funded basic science Department that is also very involved in medical student teaching. Dr. Scope is Chair of a large, very busy clinical Department responsible for a significant portion of the clinical revenues of both the hospital and the clinical faculty practice plan. With the major uncertainties of the Affordable Care Act and evolving changes at the National Institutes of Health, the Senior Leadership of the AHC is very concerned about remaining financially viable unless major changes are put in place. The Senior Leadership has requested the two Chairs join the Senior Leadership ex officio, Drs. Basic and Scope to represent and speak for respectively the research and clinical interests of all the AHC faculty; Senior Leadership intends to develop contrasting SWOT plans making the cases for versus against the following four alternatives: a) maintaining research, clinical, and educational viability with a projected 30 percent budget decrease; b) possible merging with a very large and well-known national clinic; c) considering buyout by a large for-profit health insurance company; d) developing a financial relationship with a large international pharmaceutical and device for-profit corporation. Senior Leadership has advised these two Chairs that each should expect to spend at least twenty hours/week on this project for an estimated six months.

Case 9:

Dr. Oops, the Chair of the large clinical Department Heal, receives a phone call in the early evening from the AHC security director requesting a meeting in the following early morning. At that morning meeting, the security director informs the Chair that one of the personnel collecting copays from patients at the time of outpatient service in Department Heal has been embezzling monies for the past three months. This has been detected by the usual audits conducted by the AHC. The Chair is obviously concerned and asks what the next steps are from the vantage point of AHC security. The security officer pauses and then informs the Dr. Oops that the alleged guilty individual is the son of Dean High, one of the senior academic officers of the University. Dean High oversees all the undergraduate educational programs. Dr. High's son, who had been unsuccessful in getting into law school, had been hired directly after graduation from another university as a favor to Dean High by Dr. Oops. Dr. Oops in his clinical practice was caring for Dean High as a patient at the time the Dean's son graduated. Dr. Oops' son is an undergraduate in the programs overseen by Dr. High. Dr. Oops' wife, an attorney, works as an in-house attorney in the Office of Counsel at the University.

CASE STUDIES

Case 10:

Dr. Gene, Chair of an excellent basic science Department, has several faculty involved in NIH-funded research, many with a significant translational component. Some of the faculty are funded, some are seeking renewal of funding, and some are seeking their first grants. The medical student curriculum has been redesigned. As a result of this curriculum redesign, her faculty are required to greatly increase teaching commitments, in preparation of educational materials, in curriculum refinement, and also in face-to-face teaching time with students. Because of hard-money Departmental assets consumed by research support, Dr. Gene has no available funds from the AHC to compensate her faculty for this increase in teaching responsibility and time. The faculty have recently met as a group with the Chair, expressing grave concerns that the increased time and effort needed to secure extramural funding is dictating a need for the faculty to radically decrease teaching time.

Case 11:

Dr. Hybrid is Chair of a clinical Department that includes basic research and several large clinical Divisions. The full-time faculty include six well-funded researchers (NIH) and modest clinical revenues yielding a barely break-even overall financial budget for the Department. The Department also has two faculty with research and clinical expertise in field Tiny. Tiny is an area, both clinical and research, of small impact in that there are few patients with this disease, thus representing an "orphan population." These two full-time faculty are the world's experts in this area. Their recent basic science results on the genes involved and secondary metabolic changes of this orphan disease suggest new novel therapies for two common clinical conditions outside of the Tiny field; if this proves to be true, the result might be very significant intellectual property and patent/license opportunities. The Department has limited "hard money" resources from the AHC. The Senior Leadership of the AHC has recently decreased hard-money budget support for all

322

Departments across the entire AHC. This same academic Department has a disproportionate responsibility for medical student education. Dr. Hybrid has a meeting with the Dean and the CEO to negotiate the Department budget.

Case 12:

A clinical Chair of Department U. Getum, Dr. I. B. Running, for some months has been conducting a national search for a new MD/PhD clinician scientist in a subspecialty area of which the national pool is very small. A superb candidate, Dr. I. M. Cool, has been identified. Due-diligence inquiries yield the information that Dr. Cool is an outstanding clinician, and she is conducting solid basic research with a large NIH grant that is current. Dr. Cool, although pleased with the primary clinical Department academic appointment as offered, is insisting on a secondary appointment in two basic science Departments. In spite of requests by Dr. Running, neither basic science Chair will agree to this until Dr. Cool has been on board at the AHC for a year or two. Dr. Cool has a spouse, Dr. Verb, who has a tenure-track academic appointment in the English Department of the University where they are now located. He does not insist on tenure, but does insist that his appointment be in the tenure track in the English Department of the University with which the AHC is connected. The Chair of the English Department, Dr. Poet, currently has no opening in a tenure track, although several faculty are older, one of whom is ill and with an increasing disability. Dr. Cool and Dr. Verb have two children of middle-school age, one very gifted and the other with special needs.

Some Items to Consider for Sample Prototype Documents
Introduction

Over the past twenty-five years, the author has had the opportunity and challenge to compose a variety of offer letters to prospective new faculty. During that time the author developed a "checklist" of items found to be helpful when creating the offer letter to new faculty. The author is not an attorney, and readers must solicit advice from the Dean and the Office of Counsel at his/her AHC as to how they wish offer letters composed for new prospective faculty recruits. Hopefully the material that follows will be of assistance in those endeavors.

Some concepts worth considering are:

1) **The offer letter** can serve as a very helpful document to enhance successful recruiting. The well-worded, accurate letter will:

   a) Summarize accurately all the negotiating discussions the Chair and AHC have had with the candidate. This letter should be factual, realistically enthusiastic, and friendly in tone.

   b) Allow the candidate to review the items and ask any additional questions and request clarification.

   c) Avoid misunderstanding by either the Chair or the new faculty member, once the new faculty member is on the faculty (see chapters 24, 26, 27, 28).

2) The offer letter should be written by the Chair in clear, ordinary language. Then, the letter should be reviewed by the Office of Counsel, not to rewrite, but to be certain that something the Chair stated in his/her terms does not have unintended legal implications. This is

far preferable to the Office of Counsel writing the document in legal language and the Chair then trying to clarify tone and intent.

3) The Office of Counsel and the Dean's Office may well wish a **standard document with terms for faculty employment to be attached to the offer letter.** This document will most likely be designed to precisely delineate legal issues, such as compliance with federal and state laws, visa information if applicable, HIPPA compliance, compliance with policies and regulations of the AHC, requirements and expectations of ethical behavior, etc. Because of the legal ramifications of this content, it is anticipated that the AHC will not want the Chair to modify this standard terms for faculty employment, unless approved by both the Dean and the Office of Counsel.

In crafting the offer letter, whether the portion written by the Chair (Appendix A) or the Standard Terms (Appendix B, should the AHC select this format), the sequence of items listed in the outlines below is not that necessarily used in the final letter text. The proper sequencing of the topics in the offer letter composed for the individual faculty recruit will be depend on the specifics in the AHC and the Department, and on the exact proposed role and expectations for that new faculty member. The items listed are intended as a checklist to be certain all the necessary items are addressed and understood by both the AHC/Department and the recuit.

1) **Appendix A:** This is the checklist of items for the Chair to consider for inclusion *in the portion of the offer letter text that is written by the Chair* to summarize all the prior discussions by the Chair with the faculty candidate. Not all items apply. The intent of this list is to remind the Chair of items he/she has discussed or should have discussed with the faculty candidate, and if discussed should be included in the offer letter text. If not discussed, the Chair may want to consider doing so if the item is relevant to that faculty recruit and certainly do so before crafting the Chair's final offer letter.

2) **Appendix B:** This is a checklist of items wisely considered to be *standard terms for all offer letters*; the Chair should review these items (or similar items) with the Dean's Office and the Office of Counsel at his/her AHC. If they agree that these items are nonnegotiable (except under extraordinary circumstances) and that these terms should be understood by all faculty, the Office of Counsel with the Dean's Office's input might want to craft a **standard document** to be attached to the offer letter delineating these items as deemed appropriate by the Chair's AHC's leadership.

There are two lists in this Appendix B indicating items that the AHC might wish to consider for the standard document, one for faculty with clinical activity, and one for faculty in basic science, translational, or clinical research. For faculty involved in both clinical care and in research, a composite of these two lists might be considered prudent. This checklist refers to items such as: the need for clinicians to maintain a license to practice medicine, research integrity, ethical behavior, compliance with visa regulations if applicable, compliance with policies and procedure documents of the AHC, etc. The author recommends that the text in the standard terms document *not* be changed by the Chair unless authorized by *both* the Dean and the Office of Counsel. The offer letter crafted by the Chair should attach the standard term document and contain a stated reference to the standard faculty document, such as "Attached to this letter is the standard document on terms for faculty employment that apply to all our faculty."

3) **Appendix C:** Items for Chair consideration when communicating with a faculty member at the time that faculty member is being considered for tenure

4) **Appendix D:** Suggested checklist of items for Chair and Department self-assessment of progress, status, and strategic planning

Appendix A: Items to Consider in Offer Letter Written by Chair to Faculty Recruit

(See also chapter 26)

Suggestions for Introductory Paragraphs

We are delighted to present you with this letter. As you know, we have had very productive discussions about the possibility for you to join our faculty at *Name of AHC* or *University*. We recognize that it is prudent for both you and our Medical Center to summarize the details of your proposed appointment, consistent with our prior discussions. If you have any questions or wish more information on any of the following, please let us know. We are very enthusiastic about your future career here with us.

Information of Proposed Academic Appointment:

1) Rank

2) Department

3) Duration, if without tenure

4) Tenure, if so proposed

5) Reference (with web link) to institutional policies on academic ranks and promotion processes and criteria

Expectations for the proposed role of the new faculty member as is applicable to that faculty recruit, including role in areas of professional activities, resources to be provided to the new faculty member,

and expectations for the faculty recruit's resulting accomplishments in the following areas:

1) Patient care

2) Research

3) Teaching

4) Community outreach

5) Administrative duties

6) Responsibility to be productive (i.e., what the new faculty member is expected to achieve)

7) Relationship of preceding activities to academic promotion and to compensation (with web links to policies and procedures for promotion and web links to compensation plan for faculty)

Mentoring:

1) Mentoring to be provided

2) Expectations in future to become a mentor for others

Some specifics for research faculty (basic science, translational, and clinical studies and trials):

1) Specify if this is a tenure-track or non tenure-track appointment

2) Hard copy or web link to policies and procedures for academic appointment, reappointment, promotion, and decisions for tenure

3) Research role and expectations

   a) Basic research

   b) Translational research

   c) Clinical trials

4) Possible collaborations with faculty in other Departments

5) Resources to be provided:

   a) Lab and/or bench space

   b) Laboratory support personnel, such as technicians

   c) Equipment

   d) Supplies

   e) Shared facilities within and outside Department

   f) Support from core facilities and biostatistics

   g) Start-up salary and support package (see following information on compensation), segmented by year, with expected grant success defined

   h) Outline support policy for professional personal expenses such as travel reimbursement for professional conferences and dues, consistent with IRS regulations and AHC policies (with web link if available)

6) Extramural grant-funding expectations, initially and then progressively increasing with time and academic promotion

7) Relationship of grant funding to salary

8) Teaching responsibilities

   a) Medical students (including lecture assignments, course work, and course design)

   b) Graduate teaching programs

   c) Postdoctoral trainees

d) Specify if these teaching responsibilities and/or committee service will be limited for the initial time of appointment in order to facilitate getting research and grant funding "up to speed"

e) Balance of teaching and research responsibilities after this initial protected time to initiate research

f) System for teaching evaluations and relationship to reappointments and promotions (hard copy or link to AHC policy document)

Some specifics for faculty with clinical responsibilities:

1) Hospital(s) and outpatient facilities for which privileges will be expected, and the proposed academic appointment that is predicated on successful completion of the credentialing processes for those clinical facilities

2) Hard copy or web link to policies and procedures for academic appointment, reappointment, promotion, and decisions for tenure

3) Total professional clinical responsibilities will be at the AHC facilities and affiliated facilities

4) Requirement for ABMS board certification consistent with the policies of these inpatient and outpatient facility policies

5) Ongoing need to maintain ABMS certification and recertification, consistent with policies of the ABMS on recertification

6) Information (hard copy or web link) on patient satisfaction and quality standards for the AHC

7) **For surgical disciplines**, the expectations for:

a) Number of days in clinics/week, and location for these

b) Number of operating room days/week, and facility for these

c) Support services, if applicable, such as physician extenders, receptionists, technicians, equipment, etc.

8) **For nonsurgical disciplines**, the expectations for:

a) Inpatient clinical responsibilities

b) Outpatient clinical responsibilities

c) "a" and "b" specifics on number of days per week, and/or months "on service," responsibilities, "on call"

d) If applicable, procedural responsibilities

9) **For both surgical and nonsurgical clinicians** include web-link information on the compensation system for faculty with clinical responsibilities and for this faculty recruit, as applicable, the expectations for clinical productivity, and how this will be measured:

a) Relative value units (RVU), with a target at the fiftieth percentile (or higher) of national standards for the specialty or subspecialty

b) Collections

c) Patient satisfaction and quality standards

d) Other metrics as used by Chair's AHC

Administrative and service responsibilities for all faculty:

1) Productively serve on committees to which appointed

2) Initial administrative opportunities

3) Duration of administrative responsibilities and assignments not connected to timing of academic appointments or reappointments

Teaching and educational responsibilities: (note that these will vary, depending on whether basic science or clinical faculty activities)

1) Medical student

2) Master and PhD candidates

3) Residents

4) Fellows

Compensation (provide hard copy or web link to compensation plan for clinicians and compensation plan for researchers; these usually will contain many of the details on the following items):

1) Start-up package

   a) Initial salary and duration before entering the compensation plan of the AHC for established faculty

   b) Office, secretarial support, technical support, etc.

   c) Space, equipment, etc., as pertinent for research or for clinical responsibilities

2) Ongoing salary after start-up package, and per the compensation plans, how this relates to clinical productivity and/or research productivity. Note that many AHCs do not provide a guaranteed salary. Many provide a base salary, with some sort of productivity incentive and an AHC citizen incentive; at progressively more AHCs this salary understanding includes the fact that salaries may increase or decrease on an annual basis, depending on the external and internal economic climate in conjunction with an assessment of the faculty member's performance and productivity.

3) Define how productivity is measured for clinicians (RVU, billings, collections, patient reviews, and/or quality measures).

4) Define how productivity is measured for research (extramural grant support, percentage of salary support from grants, etc., and how these change with time and academic rank).

5) Compensation, if any, for administrative and service assignments

6) Extra compensation system, if such exists

7) For clinicians, policy on accounts receivable

8) Benefits package and how this is structured (provide hard copy or web link, and provide name and phone number for the benefits office for the faculty recruit to contact)

   a) Health insurance

   b) Disability insurance

   c) Liability insurance (if clinical activity is expected)

   d) Moving expenses

   e) Vacation policies

   f) Professional travel policies

9) Intellectual property, royalties, honoraria

Closing paragraphs:

1) Refer to standard faculty terms. (The Chair needs to understand that these are best crafted by the Dean's Office and the Office of Counsel, and the Chair cannot change the attached standard document unless approved by the Dean and the Office of Counsel.)

2) Indicate that the cosignature of agreement by the faculty recruit of the letter will allow the Chair to proceed to obtain the academic appointment, via the procedures in place for that AHC.

3) Finally, a paragraph such as:

   a) On behalf of the Department/Center of _____, I

   b) Look forward to many years of professional collaboration and productivity.

c) Value of this new faculty to Department, AHC, community

d) Let me know if you have any questions

e) Sending two copies of letter

    i) No questions, sign one copy and return; keep other copy for your personal use

f) Enthusiastically welcome you to our University and/or AHC

Signatures on behalf of the AHCs:

1) The Chair

2) Other Chair(s) if there are proposed secondary appointments

3) Depending on policies of the AHC, and the specific nature of the recruiting package, other signatures may include the Dean, the Hospital Director, the individual in charge of the Faculty Compensation Plan, and/or the CEO.

Appendix B: Items to Consider for Standard Terms of Faculty Employment

(See also chapter 26)

For Faculty Involved in Clinical Care:

External regulatory expectations for faculty regarding each of the following items:

1) Completion and maintenance of hospital credentialing processes with external agencies and bodies

2) Maintenance of state medical licensure

3) Maintenance of unrestricted DEA number

4) Maintenance of participation on the local, regional, and national third-party insurance panels

5) Maintenance of appropriate specialty and subspecialty Board credentials and recertifications from the ABMS (or comparable Osteopathic body)

6) Comply with continuing medical education (CME) policies of the AHC

7) Just as the initial academic appointment is contingent upon the credentialing just referenced by the hospital(s) and state medical licensure and maintenance of the hospital appointment(s) in good standing, subsequent behavior or charges causing a faculty member to have one or more of these suspended or revoked will cause this academic appointment to be suspended or revoked.

8) If applicable, the responsibility of the faculty member to obtain and to maintain the appropriate visa and other related documents authorizing work in the United States.

    a) Throughout the term of employment

    b) Failure to do so will be grounds for immediate termination of compensation, employment, and faculty appointment.

    c) The academic Department office (or Dean's Office, depending on the AHC structure) can if you request

        i) Provide the name(s) and phone number(s) of those at AHC who can advise

9) Compliance with public health policies of the AHC, such as TB testing, immunizations

10) Compliance with illegal-drug-screening policies and procedures (hard copy attached or web link provided)

    a) Details will vary from one AHC to another.

        i) Some will do only preemployment screening

        ii) Some may repeat at intervals

        iii) Some may repeat, only for cause

    b) At most AHCs doing this testing, failure of preemployment testing for use of illegal drugs will result in the academic appointment not being recommended, and may result in reporting to appropriate oversight authorities

    c) Standards are in place to validate collection process, accommodate prescription medications, etc.

Internal regulatory expectations for Faculty:

1) Collegial and professional conduct

2) Web links listed here to all the policies of the AHC, including faculty regulations, promotion policies and procedures, conflict-of-interest policies, institutional research review board procedures, research administration policies, intellectual property and technology transfer policies, faculty compensation plan documents and policies, hospital(s) bylaws, business code of conduct

3) Consulting

   a) Web links to relevant faculty and AHC policies

   b) Result of the consulting should be of benefit to the AHC and to the faculty member's reputation

   c) Obligation to discuss with Chair before consulting

   d) Define for the faculty member the time limits for this, such as one day a week

   e) The need to avoid conflict of commitment and no loss of productivity in teaching, research, and/or clinical responsibilities at the AHC. The commitment and productivity are as defined by the Chair.

   f) Need for compliance with all conflict-of-interest and technology-transfer policies of the AHC

Productivity expectations for those with unlimited tenure:

Note that the relationship of tenure and salary is evolving at many AHCs. At the time this book was written, in more than half of AHCs tenure did not guarantee a salary level. The reader needs to collaborate with Senior Leadership and the Office of Counsel to understand the policy and practice at his/her AHC.

Should tenure not be linked to salary, the following points might be of interest to the Senior Leadership and Office of Counsel at his/her AHC when crafting the standard terms for faculty offer letters at that AHC:

1) Tenure is granted in acknowledgement of past and current academic achievement, with the understanding that productivity and AHC citizenship expectations will continue on the current upward trajectory.

2) Performance and salary will be reviewed every one, two, three years

3) At time of review, productivity and performance will determine if salary and/or other resources will increase or decrease

Consulting by faculty:

1) Intent is for the benefit of the AHC and the individual faculty

2) Web link to AHC policies on consulting

3) Web links to conflict-of-interest and technology-transfer policies as applicable to consulting

4) Need to discuss with and get approval of Chair before proceeding

5) Consulting must not interfere with time commitment to, and productivity for, the AHC and Department in clinical, research, and teaching targets. These targets are determined by the Chair.

6) Failure to meet productivity expectations or time commitments for the AHC and Department may cause decrease in faculty compensation.

Noncompete considerations:

For clinicians, both those within AHCs and those in other nonacademic situations, noncompete wording in employment documents is becoming more common. However, this is a complex legal issue with many ramifications.

Because noncompete wording is becoming more common, the Chair should collaborate with Senior Leadership and the Office of Counsel at his/her AHC. If such noncompete wording already exists for that AHC, it should be included as part of the standard faculty terms document that is attached to the Chair letter.

Should the AHC be considering the development of noncompete employment agreements with faculty, considerations include:

1) Duration or the number of years before the departing faculty member can practice clinical medicine in the area of the AHC

2) Proximity or how wide a perimeter in miles around the AHC is precluded from clinical practice during the preceding-referenced time duration

3) The preceding will apply whether the exiting faculty member is planning solo practice, or in a group, or in some type of employment with an institution

4) The decision will also need to be made as to whether or not to preclude hiring of personnel away from the AHC to the new location

5) Other clauses deemed necessary to include by Senior Leadership and the AHC's Office of Counsel and/or other legal consultants

Other legal issues:

1) Need to comply with federal, state, and local laws

2) Compliance with HIPAA

3) Criminal activity as a cause for dismissal and tenure revocation

4) AHC insists on high standards for professional and ethical behavior

5) Language specific to the AHC and the state and federal governments as to the obligations of the faculty member to notify the AHC of any action(s) against the faculty member from federal, state, or local agencies—presently or in the future—including personal issues, clinical activity, or research activity

6) This offer letter and these standard terms are the only employment agreement with the AHC and supersede all prior written or oral agreement

For Faculty Involved in Research:

External regulatory expectations for faculty:

1) Compliance with TB testing, immunization requirements, and other public health measures

2) Compliance with drug-testing policies of the AHC (provide web link or hard copy)

3) Failure of preemployment testing for use of illegal drugs will result in the academic appointment not being recommended, and may result in reporting to appropriate oversight authorities

4) If applicable, the responsibility of the faculty member to obtain and to maintain the appropriate visa and other related documents authorizing work in the United States

   a) Throughout the term of employment

   b) Failure to do so will be grounds for immediate termination of compensation, employment, and faculty appointment

   c) The academic Department office can if you request

      i) Provide the name(s) and phone number(s) of those at AHC who can advise

Internal regulatory expectations for faculty:

1) Collegial, collaborative, and professional environment

2) Website documents referenced with links for: regulations and policies and procedures for faculty; appointment, reappointment, promotion, and tenure regulations and procedures; conflict-of-interest policies; research-administration policies; intellectual and technology-transfer policies; business code of conduct; human-resource policies;

policies on ethical animal use; and radiation safety and biohazard rules and regulations.

Consulting by faculty:

1) Intent is for the benefit of the AHC and the individual faculty

2) Web link to AHC policies on consulting

3) Web links to conflict-of-interest and technology-transfer policies as applicable to consulting

4) Need to discuss with and get approval of Chair before proceeding

5) Consulting must not interfere with time commitment to, and productivity for, the AHC and Department in research and teaching targets. These targets are determined by the Chair.

6) Failure to meet productivity expectations or time commitments for the AHC and Department may cause decrease in faculty compensation.

Productivity expectations for those with unlimited tenure:

Note that the relationship of tenure and salary is evolving at AHCs. At the time this book was written, in more than half of AHCs tenure did not guarantee a salary level. The reader needs to collaborate with Senior Leadership and the Office of Counsel to understand the policy and practice at his/her AHC.

Should tenure not be linked to salary, the following points might be of interest to the Senior Leadership and Office of Counsel at his/her AHC when crafting the standard terms for faculty at that AHC:

1) Tenure is granted in acknowledgement of past and current academic achievement, with the understanding that productivity and AHC citizenship expectations will continue on the current upward trajectory.

2) Performance and salary will be reviewed every one, two, or three years

3) At time of review, productivity and performance will determine if salary and/or other resources will increase or decrease

Other Legal Items for Faculty:

1) Comply with federal, state, and local laws

2) Comply with HIPPA

3) Criminal activity is cause for dismal and loss of tenure revocation

4) Must notify the AHC and Chair if: current or future loss of eligibility for federal grants, contracts, programs; criminal activity (other than minor traffic violation); any investigation or proceedings relating to his/her research

11) This offer letter with the attached standard terms supersedes all prior written or oral agreements regarding the AHC employment

Appendix C: Suggested Items for Letter to Faculty Member Who Will Be Proposed for Promotion to Tenure

Should the AHC policy be that tenure does not guarantee any particular salary level, the following points might be considered by the Dean and the Office of Counsel in discussions with the Chair. A letter might be wise, sent to the faculty member before the institutional evaluation for tenure as proposed by the Department and Chair. This letter most likely will be signed by the appropriate individual in the Dean's Office.

Possible points for this letter are:

1) Congratulations on career to date, acknowledging success

2) Intent of letter is to clarify specifications of tenure at this AHC

3) Emphasize that tenure is considered based on academic successes and productivity in past and at present

4) Emphasize that if tenure is granted, it is with the assumption that the career trajectory will continue with the academic productivity, achievement, and with the outstanding AHC citizenship

5) Academic performance and achievements will be reviewed every one, two, or three years

6) Compensation and resources may increase or decrease consistent with demonstrated academic productivity and AHC citizenship

7) Because of enthusiasm and acknowledgement of accomplishments, the Department and the Chair are working with the faculty member to assemble the necessary supporting documents to commence the consideration for tenure according to the policies for such at this AHC.

Appendix D: Suggested Checklist of Items for Chair and Department Self-Assessment of Progress, Status, and Strategic Planning

Department Chair/Center Director's Narrative

Executive summary

1) Objectives, mission and vision, opportunities

2) Governance and organizational structure/chart

3) Areas of excellence/major accomplishments

4) Barriers to success

5) Opportunities over the next five years

Clinical Activities

1) Clinical services/organization

    a) Quality and volume: Department as a whole and subspecialty units, expressed both as totals and for individual faculty members for:

        i) Number of patients seen both new and in follow-up

        ii) RVU's of activity

        iii) Number of days from call for outpatient appointment to date patient seen

        iv) Number of inpatient consults

        v) Number of days in accounts receivable

b) Numbers and kinds of clinical procedures

c) Growth/regression of services

2) New programs

a) Relationship to hospital initiatives and goals

b) Relationship to activities and needs of other Departments

3) Financial performance of practice(s)

4) Constraints and resource availability

Research Activities

1) Description of research efforts

a) Quality and volume

b) NIH research grants and contracts

c) NIH training grants

d) Other federal grants, such as Department of Defense

e) Industry-sponsored research grants

f) Trials

2) Other funded and non-funded research

3) Trends in peer-reviewed and total support

4) Space and other resource utilization (for example, number of dollars of extramural research per square foot of space)

5) Novel research programs

Educational and Fellowship Activities

1) Medical student teaching

   a) Include student evaluation of clinical clerkship or basic science course if applicable

2) Residency/fellowship training programs

   a) Match results

      i) Current status of graduates

   b) Academic productivity by residents

      i) Research papers published (clinical or basic science refereed journals)

      ii) Prodium presentations at national academic meetings

      iii) Theses

   c) Include results of most recent RRC review

   d) Results of graduates of residency program when taking the subsequent certification examinations of the respective Board(s)

3) Continuing Medical Education

   a) Number and kind of courses taught

   b) Faculty involved and number of attendees

Community outreach

1) Health clinics (e.g., for uninsured, homeless, drug-treatment programs, free cancer screening, etc.)

2) Educational programs (e.g., public and population health education, science educational programs in local schools)

3) Outreach to other health providers (e.g., high school sport coaches and trainers, emergency medical technicians in ambulance services, collaboration with emergency responders from fire Departments, etc.)

Leadership/Administration

1) Department/Center organizational structure and organization chart

2) Faculty issues

    a) Mentoring programs for trainees and junior faculty

    b) Faculty development/retention

    c) Recruitment efforts, appointments, and promotions

    d) Diversity data: faculty and trainees

3) Process for decision making

4) Communication with faculty

Department/Center Finances: Annual and Five-Year Total

1) Income: Total

    a) Clinical income (gross and net; days in receivables)

    b) Research support (direct and indirect)

    c) Hospital support

    d) Medical School support

    e) Revenues from practice plan, as applicable

    f) Endowment income

    g) Intellectual property, patents

2) Expenses: Total

    a) Salaries and fringe

b) Incentive compensation

c) Operating expenses

d) Research overhead

e) Capital expenses

Resources

1) Space

a) Research space

b) External dollars/square foot

2) Clinical space

3) Administrative space

4) Major equipment

Fund-Raising/Marketing/PR/Endowments

1) Patents/royalties, etc.

2) Current endowments

3) New endowments

4) Income to Department from endowments

Strategic Plans

Include prior internal review(s), annual reports, and results of Departmental/center "retreat/advances"

Appendices

1) NIH biosketch or equivalent two-page CV summary of each full-time faculty member, including five most recent publications

2) Other pertinent materials/exhibits

Index

INDEX

Selected Bibliography*

1) Ambros, L. *A Mentor's Companion*. Chicago: Perrone-Ambrose Associates Inc. 1998.

2) Biebuyck, J F; Mallon, W. T. *The Successful Medical School Department Chair—a Guide to Good Institutional Practice*. Washington, DC: Association of American Medical Colleges. 2002.

3) Bledstein, B. J. *The Culture of Professionalism*. Kettering Review 1994; 31–37.

4) Boorstin, D. *The Americans: the Colonial Experience*. New York: Vintage Books 1958; 191–205.

5) Cohen, J. "Unions Are Bad Medicine for Doctors." *Chicago Tribune*, July 25, 1999.

6) Collins, J. *Good to Great: Why Some Companies Make the Leap...and Others Don't*. New York: HarperCollins. 2001.

7) Cote, D. "Whiners, Know-It-Alls and Steamrollers! Working with People Who Drive You Crazy." *Psychology Today*. ptotoday. com/0803whiner.html. Retrieved October 13, 2005.

8) D'Ambrosia, R D. "Physicians Must Put Patients First in Partnerships to Rebuild Trust." *AAOS Bulletin* 1999; April: 47.

9) Fisher, R; Ury, W, with Patton, B. *Getting to Yes—Negotiating Agreement Without Giving In*. New York: Penguin Books 2nd ed. 1991 (1st edition 1981).

10) Flexner, A. *"Is Social Work a Profession?" in W. Metzger. What is a Profession?* College and University 1976; (52): 42–55.

11) Freidson, E. *Professionalism Reborn*. Chicago: University of Chicago Press. 1994; 168–172.

12) Gaylin, W. "Faulty Diagnosis: Why Clinton's Health-Care Plan Won't Cure What Ails Us." *Harper's Magazine* 1993; October: 57–64.

13) Geisel, T. S. *Yertle the Turtle*. New York: Random House Children's Division, 1958.

14) Goleman, D. *Emotional Intelligence: Why It Can Matter More Than IQ*. New York: Bantam Books (Random House). 1995.

15) Goleman, D. "What Makes a Leader?" *Harvard Business Rev* 1998; 76 (6): 93–102.

16) Goleman, D; Boyatzis, R; McKee, A. *Primal Leadership: The Hidden Driver of Great Performance*. Boston: Harvard Business School Press. 2001.

17) Hammond, P. B.; Morgan, H. P.; eds. *Ending Mandatory Retirement for Tenured Faculty—the Consequences for Higher Education*. Commission on Behavioral and Social Sciences and Education. National Research Council. Washington, DC: National Academy Press. 1991.

18) Harari, O. *The Leadership Secrets of Colin Powell*. New York: McGraw-Hill. 2002.

19) Hecht, I. W. D.; Higgerson, M. L.; Gmelch, W. H.; Tucker, A. *The Department Chair as Academic Leader* (American Council on Education/ Oryx Press Series on Higher Education). Phoenix: Oryx Press. 1999.

20) Kappus, E. A. *Personal Communication*.

21) Kumar, S.; Nash D. B. *Demand Better—Revive Our Broken Healthcare System*. Bozeman: Second River Healthcare Press. 2011.

22) Mace, S. *Health Leaders Magazine*. www.healthleadersmedia.com. Accessed September 2012.

23) Magee M. *Health Politics—Power, Populism and Health.* Bronxville: Spencer Books. 2005.

24) McArthur, J. H.; Moore, F. D. *The Two Cultures and the Health Care Revolution.* JAMA 1997; 277(12): 985–989.

25) McCullough, N. C. *Of Geese and Golden Eggs. JBJS* 1999; 81: 303–305.

26) Peabody, F. W. *The Care of the Patient. JAMA* 1927; 88: 877–882.

27) Perlow, L. A. *Sleeping with Your Smartphone—How to Break the 24/7 Habit and Change the Way You Work.* Boston: Harvard Business Review Press. 2012.

28) Rhoades, A; Shepherdson, N. *Built on Values—Creating an Enviable Culture That Outperforms the Competition.* San Francisco: Jossey-Bass. 2011.

29) Rosenbaum, M. *Six Tires and No Plan—The Impossible Journey of the Most Inspirational Leader That (Almost) Nobody Knows.* Austin: Greenleaf Book Group Press. 2012.

30) Rothblatt, S. "How 'Professional' are the Professions?" A review article. *Comparative Studies in Society and History* 1995;37(1):194–204.

31) Rumsfeld, D. *Rumsfeld's Rules: Leadership Lessons in Business, Politics, War and Life.* New York: Broadside Books, HarperCollins Publishing. 2013.

32) Schlossberg, N. *Retire Smart, Retire Happy: Finding Your True Path in Life.* Washington, DC: American Psychological Assoc. 2003.

33) Schlossberg, N. *Revitalizing Retirement: Reshaping Your Identity, Relationships, and Purpose.* Washington, DC: American Psychological Assoc. 2009.

34) Schultz, H.; Gordon, J. *Onward—How Starbucks Fought for its Life Without Losing Its Soul.* New York: Rodale, Inc. 2011.

35) Sedlar, J.; Miners, R. *Don't Retire, Rewire!—5 Steps to Fulfilling Work That Fuels Your Passion, Suits Your Personality, and Fills Your Pocket* 2nd ed. New York: Alpha Books, Penguin Group (USA). 2007.

36) Sharp, I.; Phillips, A. *Four Seasons—The Story of a Business Philosophy.* New York: Penguin Group. 2009.

37) Sheldon, G. F. *Professionalism, Managed Care, and the Human Rights Movement. Bulletin of the American College of Surgeons* 1999; Dec:14–33.

38) Strauss, M. B., ed. *Familiar Medical Quotations.* Boston: Little Brown and Co. 1977.

39) Studer, Q. *Hardwiring Excellence: Purpose, Worthwhile Work, Making a Difference.* Gulf Bridge: Studer Group, LLC. Fire Starter Publishing. 2003.

40) Sullenberger, C.; Century, D. *Making a Difference—Stories of Vision and Courage from America's Leaders.* New York: HarperCollins. 2012.

41) Swenson, R. A. *Margin: Restoring Emotional, Physical, Financial, and Time Reserves to Overloaded Lives.* Colorado Springs: NavPress. 2004.

42) Wesberry, J. *Pursuit of Professionalism. Internal Auditor* 1989; 46(2)22–29.

43) Willmon, W. *Clergy Ethics: Getting Our Story Straight.* Goldberg, M. (ed): *Against the Grain: A New Approach to Ethics.* Harrisburg: Trinity Press Intl., 1992.

44) Wooden, J., with Jamison, S. *A Lifetime of Observations and Reflections on and off the Court.* New York: McGraw-Hill, 1997.

45) Woolhaandler, S.; Himmelstein, D. U. *When Money is the Mission— The High Costs of Investor-Owned Care. NEJM* 1999; 341: 444–46.

*This list of forty-five references is *not* to be considered inclusive, as the literature on leadership and on professionalism is huge; this list is intended only as a helpful sampling. The author has found these sources particularly interesting.

36325826R00215

Made in the USA
Lexington, KY
14 October 2014